This book is dedicated to all of the participants in our South Asian focused research studies. Thank you for giving your time to help us improve the health of all.

Introduction
The Story of my Grandfather

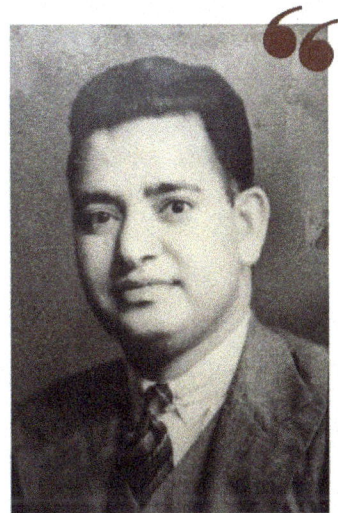

> My own grandfather's story is probably common to many others. He was taken early at the prime of his life of a sudden unexpected heart attack at age 54 years. His sudden death brought grief and sorrow, as well as concern in the family as he was the sole breadwinner.
>
> Looking back with my research lens I am struck by the intergenerational differences in risk factors and heart disease in my family.

My mother had only just made the long trip to move to and settle in Canada with her new family to begin her practice as a family doctor, when four days after she arrived, she received word that her father had suddenly passed away. She returned, flying on multiple small airplanes from rural Nova Scotia back to Uganda for her father's funeral. Looking back with my research lens I am struck by the intergenerational differences in risk factors and heart disease in my family.

> MY GRANDFATHER'S STORY IS A CLASSIC EXAMPLE OF THE SAME SEED (REPRESENTING THE GENES) RESPONDING DIFFERENTLY TO A NEW SOIL OR "ENVIRONMENT" (I.E., LIFESTYLE FACTORS LIKE DIETARY INTAKE) THAT UNEXPECTEDLY, AND NEGATIVELY INFLUENCED HIS HEALTH.

Why do I say this? What makes me conclude this? And how can three decades of research help others in their quest for optimal health for themselves and their family members? We are all taught that "an ounce of prevention is worth a pound of cure". We all wish when we have lost a loved one that we could turn back the hands of time and find that before they were stricken with disease that we could have known how to prevent the disease from happening.

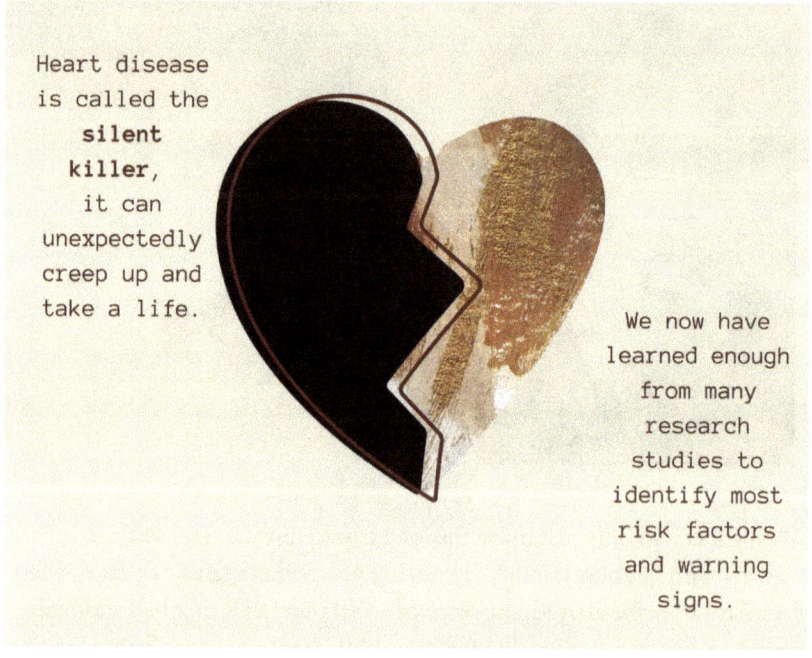

Heart disease is called the **silent killer**, it can unexpectedly creep up and take a life. We now have learned enough from many research studies to identify most risk factors and warning signs.

In my own family's story, my maternal great grandparents were born and raised in north India region of Punjab, in a small village bordering what is now Pakistan. From the village in which my Mother was born came her father and her grandparents. My Mother was raised by her grandparents and had a unique vantage point of reflecting at the end of her life - on the simplicity of their lives. She described to me how her grandmother who she called Ma, would take fresh grains, pulses, and flour to make food daily from scratch. Ma would make extra in case villagers would be without food and would drop in to share food with her family. My Mother also described being able to climb up trees and pick tropical fruits such as mangoes to eat whenever she desired. She talked about the luxury of occasionally having 'access to butter' to add to daal and to chapati's, but this was a rarity. My auntie added that Ma's sons were raised on "milk and butter". In Punjab, the milk referred to breastfeeding which continued sometimes up until age 5 years! A photograph shows my great grandparents as elders living into their 80s and thin! There was no automation in their day to day lives, and cooking took several hours each day, grinding flour, rolling chapatis, and going to their small garden, walking throughout the village to acquire foods. No energy saving devices were present in the 1930s and 40s.

When my grandfather completed his college training as a teacher, he moved to East Africa to Kampala, Uganda and became a school principal – the family celebrated as this was a sign of upward mobility! He had a good job which paid well, and he could now begin to buy more than just food, he was able to purchase the first car in the family, and he began to smoke cigarettes. When I look at pictures of him sitting in his brand-new shiny car with such a huge smile on his face, it is endearing, yet I also can see his upward mobility was reflected in his chubby face and expansive waistline. He had married for a second time a woman who was a fabulous cook, and his love of her food was reflected as excess fat in his chubby face and central fat. I surmise that this combination of central adiposity, reduced walking because he could drive his car, and cigarette smoking conspired within his arteries to lead to his sudden heart attack. I also know sadly that his brother dropped dead on the dance floor due to a heart attack age 47, living a similar lifestyle, and sadly leaving behind his wife and three daughters. So, within one generation the risk of death from heart disease before the age of 60 years went from 0 to 100%, from my great grandparents in northern India living into their late eighties, to my grandfather and his brother dying prematurely of heart disease. What accounted for this difference? Likely the substantial change in risk reflected their extreme lifestyle changes that came with upward mobility reflected in their economic comfort, labour saving devices, and adoption of new habits such as driving and cigarette smoking. This example illustrates that the same seed planted in a different soil can result in a "plant" which has reduced survival or failure to thrive.

My Mother lived in an even different soil from her Father eventually settling in rural Canada in 1965 from the age of 35 years. She lived until 84 years of age, and thankfully never suffered heart disease, stroke, or other vascular disease that we know of. She did however unfortunately acquire two different types of cancer: colon and breast cancer at two different time periods in her life: age 60 and in her late 70s respectively, to which she

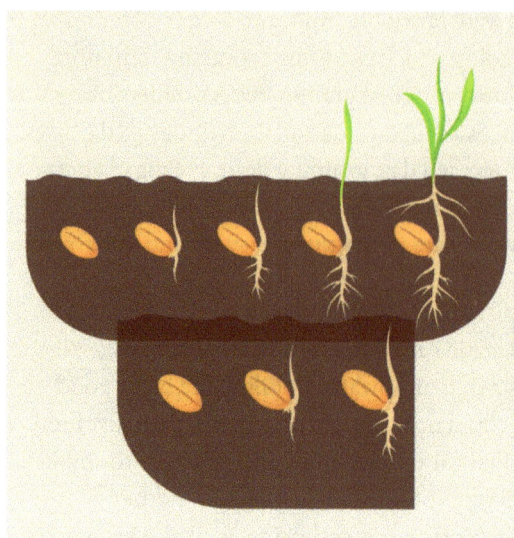

The same seed planted in a different soil can result in a "plant" which has *reduced survival or failure to thrive.*

ultimately succumbed. Again, a different soil, a different set of diseases, yet some common lifestyle features to my grandfather: little physical activity, motor vehicle transportation and more exposure to ultra-processed foods in Westernized country, although not wholly, as My Mother remained vegetarian and her traditional foods remained her common staples and her favourites lifelong. My Mother also had central adiposity and was relatively sedentary - two factors which are linked colon and breast cancer. Again, comparing my Mother to her grandparents, body fat seemed to be very different, activity and diet patterns and certainly social patterns and stressors were very different - some of these features are modifiable, others are not. One of the key features observed in most South Asian health studies is what is known as "the thin-fat phenotype" referring to the phenomenon of South Asians who are typically "normal weight" by European standards yet have fat tissue typically deposited centrally – which is associated with high levels of cholesterol, blood pressure, blood sugar, and inflammation - all of which can affect heart and brain function and has been associated with some cancers.

Chapter 1

Ancient India Texts and early observtions of Asian Indians predilection to coronary heart disease

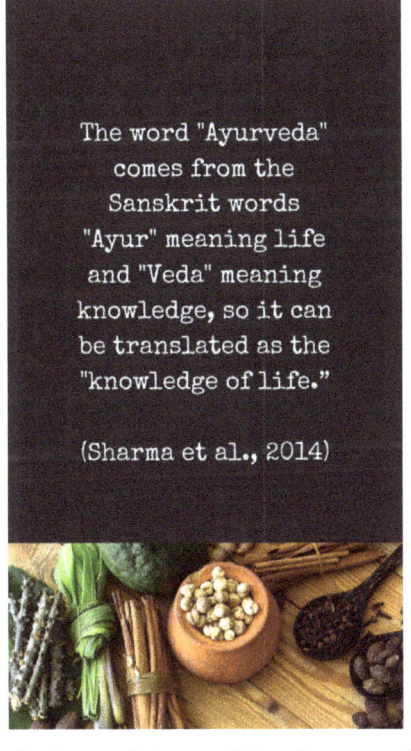

> The word "Ayurveda" comes from the Sanskrit words "Ayur" meaning life and "Veda" meaning knowledge, so it can be translated as the "knowledge of life."
>
> (Sharma et al., 2014)

Recently, I was preparing for a lifetime achievement award lecture in which I was asked to describe my research observations among South Asians with respect to diabetes. I thought I would use this opportunity to show how far we have come in our understanding of the causes of and treatments for type 2 diabetes. As a starting point, I researched to find the first mention of "sugar" and health in the classical medical texts of India or the Compendium of Charaka called the Charaka Saṃhitā, written prior to the 2nd Century. In doing so, I became engrossed in reading the Sanskrit to English translation written by PV Sharma in 1981. To my amazement it revealed the health knowledge from Ayurveda. Ayurveda is a traditional system of medicine that originated in India more than 3,000 years ago.

The scriptures I had encountered dated from as far back as the ancient Rig and Atharva Vedas (around 5000 BC) which mentioned health and diseases including phrases such as 'passing of excessive urine' which occurs with the occurrence of diabetes (Yakshma Nashana Suktam, 5th verse). Incredibly, the knowledge in this Indian system of Medicine linked "foods" to health, and even recommended a multidisciplinary team of health practitioners to care for patients with this condition called "Madhumeha" (Guddoye & Vyas, 2013; Pitta et al., 2014; Prasad et al., 2006).

Madhumeha is a disorder resembling diabetes described in the Charaka Samhita, and thought to be influenced by foods, and reduced physical activity, specifically indicating that Madhumeha was caused by: "Eating of heavy unctuous (rich in fats & oils), sour and saline substances, new grains and sweet juices in excessive amounts along with oversleeping, little exercise, neglect in evacuation" (Shree Gulabkunverba Ayurvedic Society, 2024). Furthermore, sections on the importance of diet, hygiene, prevention, medical education, the teamwork of a physician, nurse and patient necessary for recovery to health, are also detailed. Further the texts outlined that habits such as sleeping during the day, lack of exercise, indulgent drinking, or a diet full of sweet, heavy, cold and fatty foods can be attributed to the over-accumulation of adipose (fat) tissue on the body (Shree Gulabkunverba Ayurvedic Society, 2024).

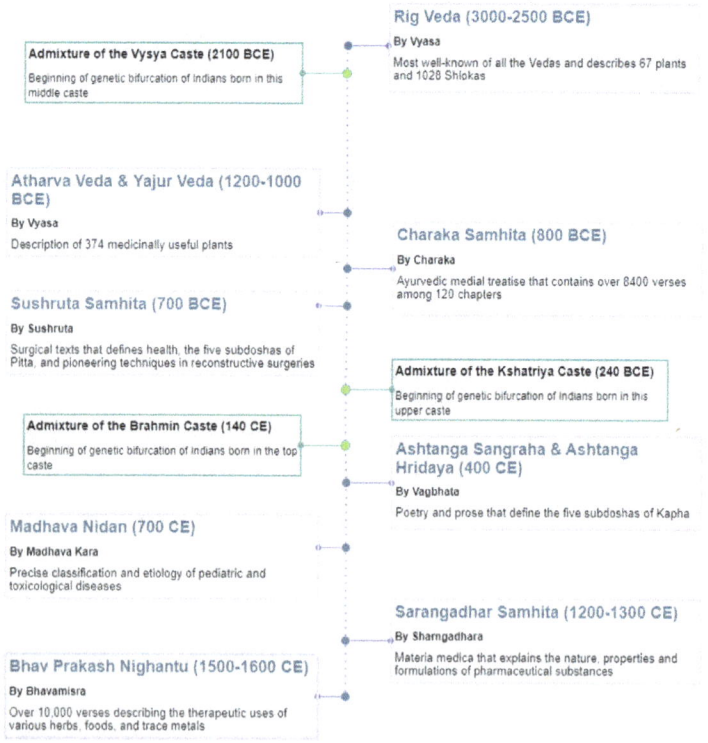

Figure 1: Timeline of the estimated creation of the central Ayurvedic corpora along with the predicted dates of inter-caste admixture (Jaiswal & Williams, 2016; Moorjani et al., 2013; Varier, 2020; Yamashita, 2018)* Prepared by Adan Amer

To my eyes, this ancient work highlighted some key components of lifestyle behaviours linked to obesity and type 2 diabetes as described in modern research studies!

The Ayurvedic medical texts described thousands of years ago some of the **common messages** we give in a clinical setting when counselling patients to prevent diabetes (Figure 1).

South Asians refer to people who originate from the Indian subcontinent including India, Pakistan, Bangladesh, Sri Lanka, Nepal, and Bhutan. In 2023 it was estimated that South Asians made up 25% of the world's population, equating to more than 2 billion people. The South Asian diaspora refers to South Asians who have left the Indian subcontinent and settled in other countries, and was estimated to be as large as 50 million people in 2023. The patterns of migration are generally dividable from the colonial phase of British rule prior to 1947, and after India gained its independence, and Pakistan was created. Pre-Independence, South Asians were sent as indentured labourers to other British colonies such as East Africa, Fiji, South Africa, and British Guyana. Post-independence others left to escape political repression, civil war, or as economic migrants to Europe, United States, Canada, and to the Middle-East (Jacobsen & Kumar, 2018). The diaspora is rich in diversity with South Asians speaking more than 30 different languages, representing diverse religions and cultural practices. As the map depicts, irrespective of the diversity from within the South Asian diaspora, there are health reports which have indicated the higher diabetes and premature heart attacks (caused by coronary artery disease) experienced by South Asians.

Interestingly just before my Grandfather's death in 1965, one of the first medical reports of early onset coronary heart disease among Asian Indians from Uganda was published in the esteemed medical journal, The Lancet. The authors remarked that coronary heart disease was very rarely observed in African men, whereas it accounted for 43% of the cases among South Asian men. (Shaper & Jones, 1959). The authors contrasted the differences in fat consumption and cholesterol measurements in the two groups. The focus on fat consumption and heart disease likely came from publications in the 1950's by Dr. Ancel Keys from the USA who promoted the dietary fat- heart disease hypothesis. In addition another study by Danaraj et al in

1959 from Singapore reported that heart disease accounted for the cause of death in 50% of South Asians compared to only 10- 20% of Chinese males over the age of 20 years, again showing South Asians propensity to develop early heart disease (Danaraj et al., 1959). Within India, Malholtra analyzed data from more than eight hundred South Asian men and women assembled from 1948-1955; and reported a seven to one male to female predominance of heart disease, the average age was 50-59 years, with the majority of men with heart disease coming from higher socioeconomic positions often having urban desk jobs (Malhotra & Pathania, 1958). These researchers found no evidence that vegetarians were immune from heart disease; and did not find convincing evidence that fat consumption in the diet played a significant role in the etiology of heart disease. The authors were struck by the propensity of heart disease that ran in families, concluding there must be 'genetic factors' at play (Malhotra & Pathania, 1958).

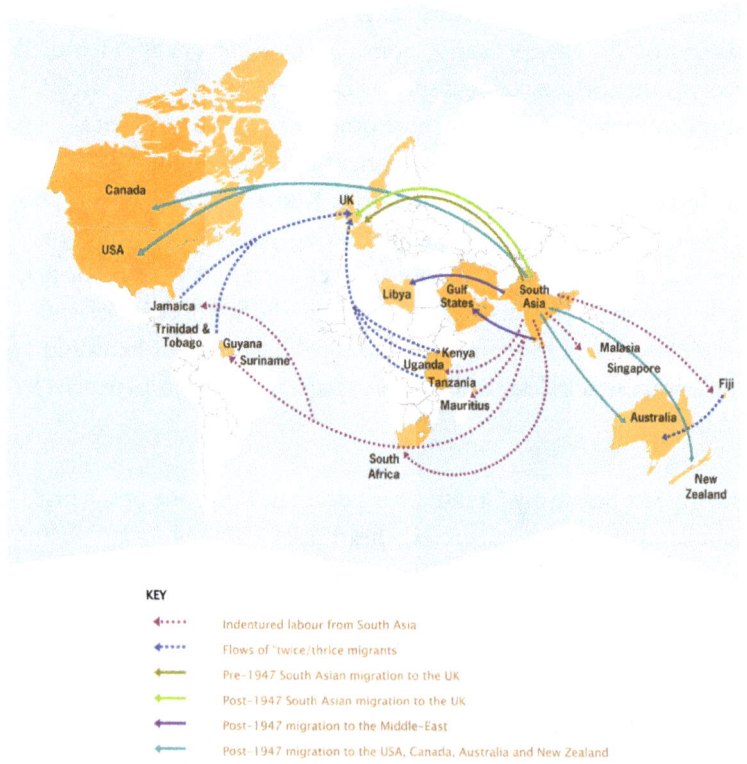

Figure 2: World Map Showing South Asian Diaspora (Map of Major South Asian Migration Flows | Reprinted from Striking Women, n.d.).

In Canada during the mid-90s, when we analyzed national databases by ethnicity, South Asians indeed had a higher risk of heart disease compared to Chinese and white Europeans (Sheth et al., 1999). We then undertook an examination of free living South Asians in Canada from three Canadian cities in the Study of Heart Assessment and Risk in Ethnic groups (SHARE) and measured a wide array of risk factors (Anand et al., 2000). In short, when compared to other ethnic groups such as people of Chinese origin and white Europeans, South Asians had a higher prevalence of the following risk factors.

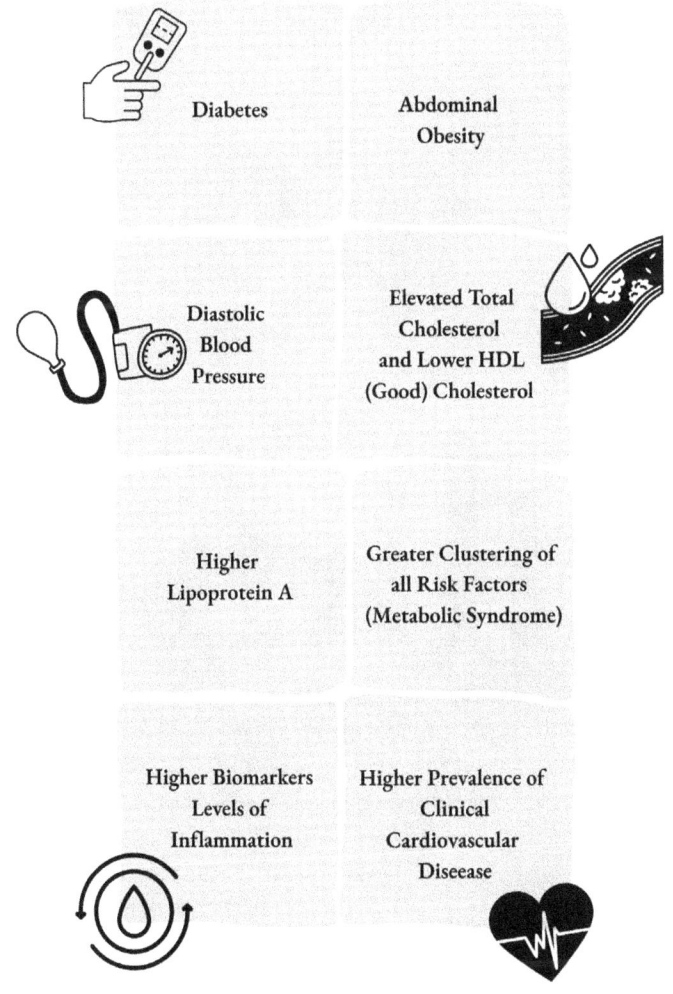

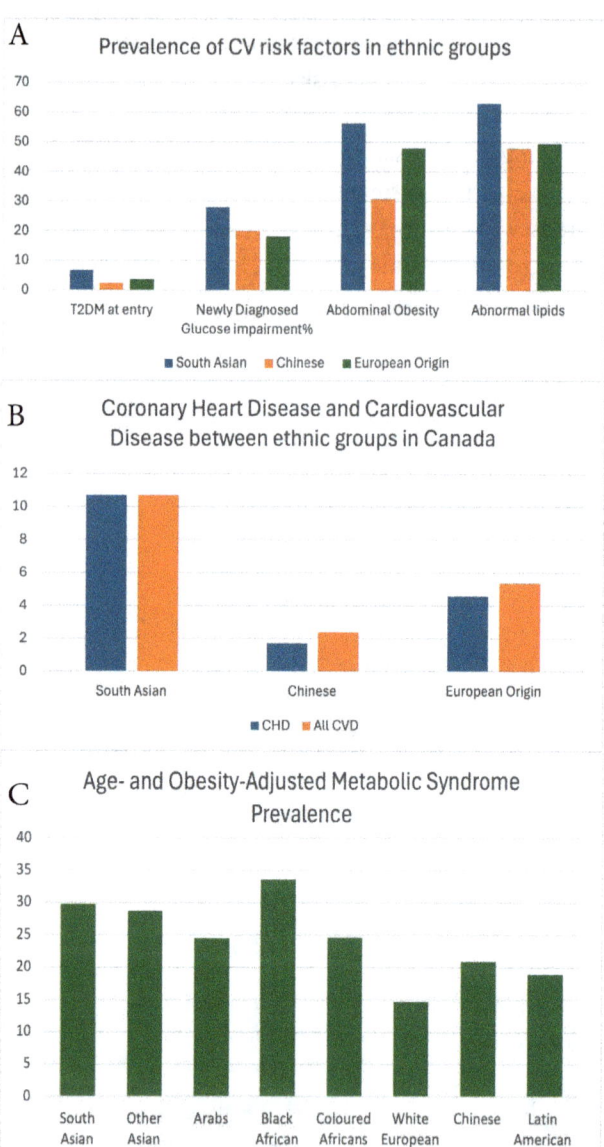

Figure 3 (A) Prevalence of type 2 diabetes and abdominal obesity in persons of South Asian, Chinese, and European origin. South Asians had the highest non-HDL cholesterol; (B) Coronary heart disease and cardiovascular disease between ethnic groups in Canada; (C) Risk of first heart attack Risk of First Heart Attack (Reprinted from Mente et al., 2010).

Note: The age- and obesity-adjusted prevalence of Metabolic Syndrome in heart attack cases was significantly higher in South Asians (29.8%, 95% CI: 27.1% to 32.5%), other Asians (28.7%, 95% CI: 24.6% to 32.8%), Arabs (25.4%, 95% CI: 22.7% to 28.1%), Black Africans (33.6%, 95% CI: 24.0% to 47.6%), and Colored Africans (24.6%, 95% CI: 18.9% to 30.3%) compared with white Europeans (14.7%, 95% CI: 12.8% to 16.6%), Chinese (20.9%, 95% CI: 19.1% to 22.7%), and Latin Americans (18.9%, 95% CI: 16.0% to 21.8%) in the INTERHEART MI Case Control Study.

The metabolic syndrome refers to a syndrome when multiple cardio-metabolic risk factors are present at the same time. The metabolic syndrome can be defined in a number of ways, but one common definition is the presence of abdominal obesity plus 2 other risk factors, such as diabetes, high blood pressure or abnormal cholesterol (Alberti et al., 2006). The metabolic syndrome is associated with a 2-fold increase in heart attack risk across all ethnic groups (Mente et al., 2010). However, because South Asians have the syndrome commonly, the world-wide impact of the metabolic syndrome in causing heart disease is amongst the highest in the world.

In a follow-up analysis of the same INTERHEART study Joshi and colleagues (2007) showed that South Asians compared to non-South Asians have an earlier onset first heart attack, which is largely explained by their higher amount of metabolic syndrome risk factors present at younger age of onset compared to non-South Asians.

When we delved more deeply to understand why the South Asian population had more risk factors, diabetes, and cardiovascular disease in a subsequent investigation in which South Asians men and women were matched to white European men and women by body mass index, we found that South Asians had more visceral adipose tissue, more fat deposited in the liver, along with elevated glucose and cholesterol, and other abnormal biomarkers associated with fat tissue excess (Anand et al., 2011).

In the coming Chapters we will revisit the genetic, dietary, and activity evidence that underlies the risk of metabolic syndrome risk factors and heart disease among South Asians. We will review early migrant studies which first highlighted the observation that people who originate from India suffered a higher prevalence of diabetes and coronary heart disease compared to other populations; next to the cutting edge research highlighting the role of genetics, and epigenetics. Finally we will bring all of the information we have accumulated from the last 5000 years, combining insights from Ayurvedic medicine, and contemporary scientific evidence, to provide guidance for you and your loved ones in the prevention of type 2 diabetes and heart disease.

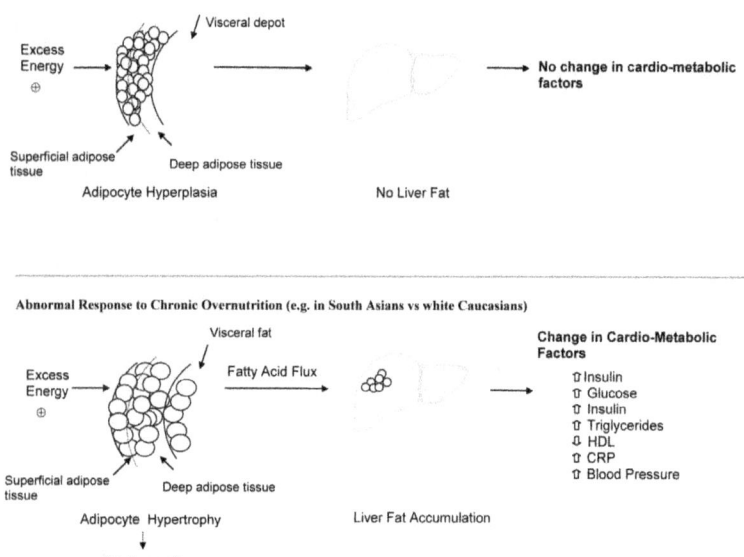

Figure 4: Mol-SHARE study South Asian Fat Tissue Excess (Reprinted from Anand et al., 2011). Note: HDL: High Density Lipoprotein, CRP: C-reactive protein.

REFERENCES

Alberti, K. G. M. M., Zimmet, P., & Shaw, J. (2006). Metabolic syndrome—A new world-wide definition. A Consensus Statement from the International Diabetes Federation. Diabetic Medicine, 23(5), 469–480. https://doi.org/10.1111/j.1464-5491.2006.01858.x

Anand, S. S., Tarnopolsky, M. A., Rashid, S., Schulze, K. M., Desai, D., Mente, A., Rao, S., Yusuf, S., Gerstein, H. C., & Sharma, A. M. (2011). Adipocyte Hypertrophy, Fatty Liver and Metabolic Risk Factors in South Asians: The Molecular Study of Health and Risk in Ethnic Groups (molSHARE). PLOS ONE, 6(7), e22112. https://doi.org/10.1371/journal.pone.0022112

Anand, S. S., Yusuf, S., Vuksan, V., Devanesen, S., Teo, K. K., Montague, P. A., Kelemen, L., Yi, C., Lonn, E., Gerstein, H., Hegele, R. A., & McQueen, M. (2000). Differences in risk factors, atherosclerosis, and cardiovascular disease between ethnic groups in Canada: The Study of Health Assessment and Risk in Ethnic groups (SHARE). Lancet (London, England), 356(9226), 279–284. https://doi.org/10.1016/s0140-6736(00)02502-2

Danaraj, T. J., Acker, M. S., Danaraj, W., Wong, H. O., & Tan, B. Y. (1959). Ethnic group differences in coronary heart disease in Singapore: An analysis of necropsy records. American Heart Journal, 58, 516–526. https://doi.org/10.1016/0002-8703(59)90085-7

Guddoye, G., & Vyas, M. (2013). Role of diet and lifestyle in the management of Madhumeha (Diabetes Mellitus). Ayu, 34(2), 167–173. https://doi.org/10.4103/0974-8520.119672

Jacobsen, K. A., & Kumar, P. (Eds.). (2018). South Asians in the Diaspora: Histories and Religious Traditions. Brill. https://brill.com/edcollbook/title/7766

Jaiswal, Y. S., & Williams, L. L. (2016). A glimpse of Ayurveda – The forgotten history and principles of Indian traditional medicine. Journal of Traditional and Complementary Medicine, 7(1), 50–53. https://doi.org/10.1016/j.jtcme.2016.02.002

Joshi, P., Islam, S., Pais, P., Reddy, S., Dorairaj, P., Kazmi, K., Pandey, M. R., Haque, S., Mendis, S., Rangarajan, S., & Yusuf, S. (2007). Risk Factors for Early Myocardial Infarction in South Asians Compared With Individuals in Other Countries. JAMA, 297(3), 286–294. https://doi.org/10.1001/jama.297.3.286

Malhotra, R. P., & Pathania, N. S. (1958). Some aetiological aspects of coronary heart disease; an Indian point of view based on a study of 867 cases seen during 1948-55. British Medical Journal, 2(5095), 528–531. https://doi.org/10.1136/bmj.2.5095.528

Map of major South Asian migration flows | Striking Women. (n.d.). Retrieved January 15, 2024, from https://www.striking-women.org/page/map-major-south-asian-migration-flows

Mente, A., Yusuf, S., Islam, S., McQueen, M. J., Tanomsup, S., Onen, C. L., Rangarajan, S., Gerstein, H. C., Anand, S. S., & INTERHEART Investigators. (2010). Metabolic syndrome and risk of acute myocardial infarction a case-control study of 26,903 subjects from 52 countries. Journal of the American College of Cardiology, 55(21), 2390–2398. https://doi.org/10.1016/j.jacc.2009.12.053

Moorjani, P., Thangaraj, K., Patterson, N., Lipson, M., Loh, P.-R., Govindaraj, P., Berger, B., Reich, D., & Singh, L. (2013). Genetic Evidence for Recent Population Mixture in India. The American Journal of Human Genetics, 93(3), 422–438. https://doi.org/10.1016/j.ajhg.2013.07.006

Pitta, S., devi, K. P., & Shailaja, B. (2014). Diabetes mellitus (Madhumeha)-an Ayurvedic review. International Journal of Pharmacy and Pharamceutical Sciences, 6.

Prasad, G. P., Babu, G., & Swamy, G. K. (2006). A contemporary scientific support on role of ancient ayurvedic diet and concepts in diabetes mellitus (madhumeha). Ancient Science of Life, 25(3–4), 84–91.

Shaper, A. G., & Jones, K. W. (1959). Serum-cholesterol, diet, and coronary heart-disease in Africans and Asians in Uganda. Lancet (London, England), 2(7102), 534–537. https://doi.org/10.1016/s0140-6736(59)91777-5

Sharma, G. K., Barthakur, M., & Sharma, R. K. (2014). Pre & post Vedic plants used in Diabetes—A database study. International Ayurvedic Medical Journal, 2(3), 350–355.

Sheth, T., Nair, C., Nargundkar, M., Anand, S., & Yusuf, S. (1999). Cardiovascular and cancer mortality among Canadians of European, south Asian and Chinese origin from 1979 to 1993: An analysis of 1.2 million deaths. CMAJ, 161(2), 132–138.

Shree Gulabkunverba Ayurvedic Society. (2024, November 30). Charaka Samhita (English translation). Wisdom Library. https://www.wisdomlib.org/hinduism/book/charaka-samhita-english

Varier, M. R. R. (2020). Early Historic Phase. In M. R. R. Varier (Ed.), A Brief History of Āyurveda (p. 0). Oxford University Press. https://doi.org/10.1093/oso/9780190121082.003.0001

Yamashita, T. (2018). Sanskrit Medical Literature. In P. T. Keyser & J. Scarborough (Eds.), Oxford Handbook of Science and Medicine in the Classical World (p. 0). Oxford University Press. https://doi.org/10.1093/oxfordhb/9780199734146.013.66

Chapter 2
The problem with South Asians
(a seed in the soil hypothesis)

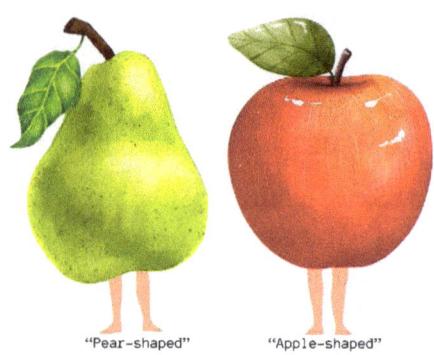

"Pear-shaped"   "Apple-shaped"

Have you ever observed at a family gathering, how some people carry their excess fat tightly around their abdominal region whereas others are generally fat all over their legs, arms, face, and hips? These two types of excess fat carriage are referred to as "Apple-Shaped" versus "Pear Shaped" fat distribution.

Well, in short South Asians are far more prone to carry excess fat tissue in an Apple-shaped distribution. Look around you – you may observe this beach ball with skinny arms and legs shape around you, or you may notice subtle trends towards this, when YOU gain weight, where the first place you notice this extra weight is with an out pouching of your tummy, and tight-fitting pants at the waist.

I have always been struck by this observation - especially when visiting India, observing low body weight men (in particular) who also have a small pot belly. These individuals are not overweight by conventional western definitions (e.g. using body mass index), and therefore typically told "they are just fine". So, is this apple shaped fat distribution of a normal weight man or women cause for concern? And if so, why is it that excess fat at all be stored around the abdomen? And why do South Asians have this more commonly than other groups?

South Asian studies have shown that a persistent multigenerational unique predilection to central adiposity and high adipose tissue to non-adipose tissue mass at birth that persists into adulthood when compared to white Europeans (Yajnik et al., 2002, 2003). We have shown this pattern exists in adults and in newborns (Anand et al., 2000; Anand, Vasudevan, et al., 2013). Another component of the South Asian phenotype is small birthweight babies with relatively more adipose tissue compared to white European babies (Anand et al., 2016). These observations provide support for a unique genetic and gene expression signature that likely exists in South Asians– reflecting ancestry and prior pregnancy and early life exposures (Anand, Vasudevan, et al., 2013).

As a researcher in this field, there are many hypotheses that have been put forth to explain this phenomenon in South Asians. Here are a few of them and the associated observations.

The Thrifty Gene hypothesis put forth by James Neel in 1962 suggested that populations exposed to feast times followed by famine times, had a genetic adaptation to enable survival famine by storing fat centrally so that it could be called upon to be utilized as fatty acids and generate glucose when glycogen supplies were depleted (Neel, 1962). However modern-day genetic studies have not confirmed this to be true (Ayub et al., 2014; Gosling et al., 2015; Steinthorsdottir et al., 2014).

Genetic Predisposition: The early case series published by Malhotra from India in the 1950 also concluded that without a doubt there was a genetic reason for the early onset coronary heart disease hereafter referred to as heart disease, the first clues provided by the strong family histories reported (Malhotra & Pathania, 1958). Genetic variants can be present in each one of the known risk factors for heart disease such as high cholesterol, diabetes, high blood pressure and abdominal obesity. South Asian studies have shown that a persistent multigenerational unique predilection to central adiposity and high adipose tissue to non-adipose tissue mass at birth that persists into adulthood when compared to white Europeans (Yajnik et al., 2002, 2003). This also raises support for a unique genetic and gene expression signature that likely exists in South Asians– reflecting ancestry and prior exposures (Anand, Vasudevan, et al., 2013). To date more than 40 genetic variants have been significantly linked to development of central fat providing solid backing to a genetic component of this common characteristic, which is not exclusive to but more common in South Asians (Herrera et al., 2011).

South Asians Genetic Propensity to risk factors for cardiovascular disease

Previous investigations have shown that South Asians have a greater frequency of genetic variants associated with gestational diabetes and type 2 diabetes (Anand, Meyre, et al., 2013; Lamri et al., 2022). When counting genetic variants for diabetes between South Asian, white Europeans and Latinos, South Asians have the higher score, and because each variants in the gene score is a predictor of future development of type 2 diabetes, South Asians are therefore higher risk of developing type 2 diabetes due to genetic factors compared to the other two ethnic groups (Anand, Meyre, et al., 2013; Mahajan et al., 2022). Specific gene variants related to insulin resistance and beta-cell function have been identified and there are complex interactions between genetic and environmental factors, such as dietary habits and physical activity levels. Many of the genetic variants associated with type 2 diabetes are also related to traits of body fat and muscle mass and cardiovascular disease (Mahajan et al., 2022).

The Caste System leads to non-random mating: Another ancestral predilection that could explain a genetic predisposition to diabetes – which we learn from ancient DNA studies. Priya Moorjani and David Reich reconstructed the Indian subcontinent populations using ancient DNA as well as information from historical social structures such as the Caste system to help us understand the history of admixture in the Indian subcontinent (Moorjani et al., 2013). They identified that there are some distinct DNA markers separating North Indians from South Indians and from those who originate from the Andaman Islands (Moorjani et al., 2013). Using ancient DNA, they reconstructed the history of migration and admixing on the Indian subcontinent, and elegantly showed how the Caste system – a social construct which prevented random mating – led to an increase in recessive alleles or so-called bottle neck populations within South Asian subpopulations (Moorjani et al., 2013). This increase in recessive alleles is associated with some health conditions like type 2 diabetes, and added to this is the cultural expectation of interfamily marriage which can increase this even

(Moorjani et al., 2013). Furthermore, in some countries far from the Indian subcontinent where South Asian migrated, they may face a double jeopardy through intermarriage within castes, as well as a closed mating population due to the remoteness of communities (e.g. Trinidad and Guyana). The increased frequency of atherosclerosis and diabetes causing genetic variants may help explain the higher burden of heart disease in parts of the South Asian diaspora.

The Thrifty Phenotype hypothesis argues that the effects of poor nutrition in early life, produces permanent changes in glucose-insulin metabolism, and places the individual at increased risk of future type 2 diabetes (Hales & Barker, 2001; A. C. J. Ravelli et al., 1998). Evidence for this hypothesis comes from populations who have faced starvation in the last century, as offspring often show evidence of the long-term effect of the stressor of famine, on their ability to store fat and their predisposition to pre-diabetes and diabetes. For example, in the Dutch Hunger Winter of World War 2, in which the Nazis closed of the food supply to the Dutch, Dutch women who were pregnant and starving had offspring who were not only smaller than expected at birth, but who were considered to have abdominal obesity and pre-diabetes were observed by the first 2 decades of their lives (Lumey et al., 2011; A. C. J. Ravelli et al., 1998; Roseboom et al., 2011) Why would this occur? The developing fetus could be thought of as a scavenger trying to compete for any calories and nutrients, such as amino acids, from the mother. They used any energy and nutrients as judiciously as possible – and these mechanisms of storing energy were hard wired into them after birth. This would stand them well if they faced nutrient shortages again, but in the scenario of energy excess (which is common in high income countries and urban areas of low-income countries), this excess energy and nutrients would result in excess abdominal adipose tissue, diabetes, and early heart disease (G. P. Ravelli et al., 1976). This supports the idea that the fetal environment can have long-lasting effects on health and highlights the importance of maternal nutrition and health during pregnancy. The insulin like growth factor 1 (IGF-1) genetic polymorphism has been implicated as being subject to epigenetic modification (Kyle & Pichard, 2006).

Epigenetics refers to marks such as methylation CPG or histone modification of genes that affect how genes are expressed, meaning how they create proteins. Environmental influences during pregnancy can mark fetal DNA and influence the "expression" of DNA as the newborns develop. These can include influences from exposure to cigarette smoking to vitamin deficiencies as part of dietary intake during pregnancy. An interesting analysis of South Asian women born in the United Kingdom, in which the birth weight of these second-generation South Asians offspring was compared to white European original citizens of UK, showed that South Asian offspring remain lower birthweight by approximately 200 grams (Leon & Moser, 2012).

The persistent lower birthweight of South Asian babies comparing India to the UK could be explained by a different seed (genetics) in a different soil (environment), but within the UK the comparison is a different seed in similar soil for the 1st generation, and in the same soil for 2nd generation offspring. To keep this analogy going, a persistent difference in how tall the plant grows in two generations is similar in identical soil and does point to a seed difference - either genetic or persistent epigenetic difference.

Thus, there are multiple theories as to why South Asians develop type 2 diabetes at higher rates than other ethnic populations – from an excess of recessive alleles as a reflection of distant migration and admixture patterns, and/or epigenetic marks reflecting past in utero exposures that influence gene expression, all of which can have different manifestations in the presence of particular health behaviors such as dietary intake and physical activity- and there are also likely other factors at play.

What about biomarkers of risk - adipokines adiponectin and leptin?

Biomarker	Role	Cardiovascular Implications
Adiponectin	Adiponectin is primarily secreted by adipose (fat) tissue It has anti-inflammatory and insulin-sensitizing properties Higher levels of adiponectin are generally associated with better metabolic health	Low levels of adiponectin have been linked to insulin resistance, inflammation, and an increased risk of cardiovascular diseases, including coronary artery disease. Adiponectin may have protective effects on the vascular system.
Leptin	Leptin is also produced by adipose tissue It is involved in regulating appetite and energy expenditure It signals to the brain to reduce food intake and increase energy expenditure	Leptin resistance, where the body becomes less responsive to the appetite-suppressing effects of leptin, has been associated with obesity. While leptin levels are generally elevated in obesity, the effectiveness of leptin signaling may be diminished. Elevated leptin levels have been linked to inflammation and may contribute to cardiovascular risk. In addition to adiponectin and leptin, other inflammatory markers may play a role in diabetes risk among South Asians. Chronic low-grade inflammation, often reflected in elevated levels of inflammatory markers, is associated with insulin resistance and the development of type 2 diabetes. South Asians may exhibit a pro-inflammatory adipokine profile.

Table 1: Biomarker roles and cardiovascular implications

Our studies indicate that South Asians have the least favorable adipokine profile and, display a greater increase in insulin resistance with decreasing levels of adiponectin. Further we have shown that South Asians in whom the metabolic syndrome is highly prevalent have higher levels of inflammatory proteins called C- Reactive protein (Mente et al., 2010).

How can I change my genetic risk?

Healthy active living is recommended to "turn off" certain genetic factors and has been shown robustly in other populations for example. We showed in a previous analysis that individuals who were born with a genetic risk of myocardial infarction or heart attack could negate this risk by consuming a diet high in fruit and vegetables (Do et al., 2011). You cannot change your genetic code, but you have some influence over minimizing the genetic risk from being transmitted to your offspring- for example, not marrying blood relatives, nor promoting only marrying strictly within a caste, are some considerations.

Anything else? This field of research is accelerating, especially as the technological advances including the ability to sequence the entire human genome with robotic technology in a short time at relatively lower cost, means we will learn a lot regarding genetic and epigenetic differences in the coming decade. In the meantime, the typical South Asian risk pattern can be summarized as such:

Knowing all this, and knowing that researchers are racing to understand why, and not being able to wait for two more decades, what can you do now to prevent you from becoming another South Asian statistic? As it is often stated, "Genetics loads the gun, and your environment pulls the trigger". That means you have the chance to prevent heart disease and diabetes by being aware and beginning your journey to health.

REFERENCES

Anand, S. S., Gupta, M. K., Schulze, K. M., Desai, D., Abdalla, N., Wahi, G., Wade, C., Scheufler, P., McDonald, S. D., Morrison, K. M., Vasudevan, A., Dwarakanath, P., Srinivasan, K., Kurpad, A., Gerstein, H. C., & Teo, K. K. (2016). What accounts for ethnic differences in newborn skinfold thickness comparing South Asians and White Caucasians? Findings from the START and FAMILY Birth Cohorts. International Journal of Obesity, 40(2), Article 2. https://doi.org/10.1038/ijo.2015.171

Anand, S. S., Meyre, D., Pare, G., Bailey, S. D., Xie, C., Zhang, X., Montpetit, A., Desai, D., Bosch, J., Mohan, V., Diaz, R., McQueen, M. J., Cordell, H. J., Keavney, B., Yusuf, S., Gaudet, D., Gerstein, H., Engert, J. C., & on behalf of the EpiDREAM Genetics Investigators. (2013). Genetic Information and the Prediction of Incident Type 2 Diabetes in a High-Risk Multiethnic Population: The EpiDREAM genetic study. Diabetes Care, 36(9), 2836–2842. https://doi.org/10.2337/dc12-2553

Anand, S. S., Vasudevan, A., Gupta, M., Morrison, K., Kurpad, A., Teo, K. K., Srinivasan, K., & The START Cohort Study Investigators. (2013). Rationale and design of South Asian Birth Cohort (START): A Canada-India collaborative study. BMC Public Health, 13(1), 79. https://doi.org/10.1186/1471-2458-13-79

Anand, S. S., Yusuf, S., Vuksan, V., Devanesen, S., Teo, K. K., Montague, P. A., Kelemen, L., Yi, C., Lonn, E., Gerstein, H., Hegele, R. A., & McQueen, M. (2000). Differences in risk factors, atherosclerosis, and cardiovascular disease between ethnic groups in Canada: The Study of Health Assessment and Risk in Ethnic groups (SHARE). Lancet (London, England), 356(9226), 279–284. https://doi.org/10.1016/s0140-6736(00)02502-2

Ayub, Q., Moutsianas, L., Chen, Y., Panoutsopoulou, K., Colonna, V., Pagani, L., Prokopenko, I., Ritchie, G. R. S., Tyler-Smith, C., McCarthy, M. I., Zeggini, E., & Xue, Y. (2014). Revisiting the thrifty gene hypothesis via 65 loci associated with susceptibility to type 2 diabetes. American Journal of Human Genetics, 94(2), 176–185. https://doi.org/10.1016/j.ajhg.2013.12.010

Do, R., Xie, C., Zhang, X., Männistö, S., Harald, K., Islam, S., Bailey, S. D., Rangarajan, S., McQueen, M. J., Diaz, R., Lisheng, L., Wang, X., Silander, K., Peltonen, L., Yusuf, S., Salomaa, V., Engert, J. C., Anand, S. S., & Investigators, on behalf of the I. (2011). The Effect of Chromosome 9p21 Variants on Cardiovascular Disease May Be Modified by Dietary Intake: Evidence from a Case/Control and a Prospective Study. PLOS Medicine, 8(10), e1001106. https://doi.org/10.1371/journal.pmed.1001106

Gosling, A. L., Buckley, H. R., Matisoo-Smith, E., & Merriman, T. R. (2015). Pacific Populations, Metabolic Disease and 'Just-So Stories': A Critique of the 'Thrifty Genotype' Hypothesis in Oceania. Annals of Human Genetics, 79(6), 470–480. https://doi.org/10.1111/ahg.12132

Hales, C. N., & Barker, D. J. P. (2001). The thrifty phenotype hypothesis: Type 2 diabetes. British Medical Bulletin, 60(1), 5–20. https://doi.org/10.1093/bmb/60.1.5

Herrera, B. M., Keildson, S., & Lindgren, C. M. (2011). Genetics and epigenetics of obesity. Maturitas, 69(1), 41–49. https://doi.org/10.1016/j.maturitas.2011.02.018

Kyle, U. G., & Pichard, C. (2006). The Dutch Famine of 1944-1945: A pathophysiological model of long-term consequences of wasting disease. Current Opinion in Clinical Nutrition and Metabolic Care, 9(4), 388–394. https://doi.org/10.1097/01.mco.0000232898.74415.42

Lamri, A., Limbachia, J., Schulze, K. M., Desai, D., Kelly, B., de Souza, R. J., Paré, G., Lawlor, D. A., Wright, J., & Anand, S. S. (2022). The genetic risk of gestational diabetes in South Asian women. eLife, 11, e81498. https://doi.org/10.7554/eLife.81498

Leon, D. A., & Moser, K. A. (2012). Low birth weight persists in South Asian babies born in England and Wales regardless of maternal country of birth. Slow pace of acculturation, physiological constraint or both? Analysis of routine data. J Epidemiol Community Health, 66(6), 544–551. https://doi.org/10.1136/jech.2010.112516

Lumey, L. H., Stein, A. D., & Susser, E. (2011). Prenatal Famine and Adult Health. Annual Review of Public Health, 32, 10.1146/annurev-publhealth-031210–101230. https://doi.org/10.1146/annurev-publhealth-031210-101230

Mahajan, A., Spracklen, C. N., Zhang, W., Ng, M. C. Y., Petty, L. E., Kitajima, H., Yu, G. Z., Rüeger, S., Speidel, L., Kim, Y. J., Horikoshi, M., Mercader, J. M., Taliun, D., Moon, S., Kwak, S.-H., Robertson, N. R., Rayner, N. W., Loh, M., Kim, B.-J., … Morris, A. P. (2022). Multi-ancestry genetic study of type 2 diabetes highlights the power of diverse populations for discovery and translation. Nature Genetics, 54(5), Article 5. https://doi.org/10.1038/s41588-022-01058-3

Malhotra, R. P., & Pathania, N. S. (1958). Some aetiological aspects of coronary heart disease; an Indian point of view based on a study of 867 cases seen during 1948-55. British Medical Journal, 2(5095), 528–531. https://doi.org/10.1136/bmj.2.5095.528

Mente, A., Razak, F., Blankenberg, S., Vuksan, V., Davis, A. D., Miller, R., Teo, K., Gerstein, H., Sharma, A. M., Yusuf, S., Anand, S. S., & for the Study of Health Assessment and Risk Evaluation (SHARE) and SHARE in Aboriginal Peoples (SHARE-AP) Investigators. (2010). Ethnic Variation in Adiponectin and Leptin Levels and Their Association With Adiposity and Insulin Resistance. Diabetes Care, 33(7), 1629–1634. https://doi.org/10.2337/dc09-1392

Moorjani, P., Thangaraj, K., Patterson, N., Lipson, M., Loh, P.-R., Govindaraj, P., Berger, B., Reich, D., & Singh, L. (2013). Genetic Evidence for Recent Population Mixture in India. The American Journal of Human Genetics, 93(3), 422–438. https://doi.org/10.1016/j.ajhg.2013.07.006

Neel, J. V. (1962). Diabetes Mellitus: A "Thrifty" Genotype Rendered Detrimental by "Progress"? American Journal of Human Genetics, 14(4), 353–362.

Ravelli, A. C. J., Meulen, J. van der, Michels, R. P. J., Osmond, C., Barker, D. J. P., Hales, C. N., & Bleker, O. P. (1998). Glucose tolerance in adults after prenatal exposure to famine. The Lancet, 351(9097), 173–177. https://doi.org/10.1016/S0140-6736(97)07244-9

Ravelli, G. P., Stein, Z. A., & Susser, M. W. (1976). Obesity in young men after famine exposure in utero and early infancy. The New England Journal of Medicine, 295(7), 349–353. https://doi.org/10.1056/NEJM197608122950701

Roseboom, T. J., Painter, R. C., van Abeelen, A. F. M., Veenendaal, M. V. E., & de Rooij, S. R. (2011). Hungry in the womb: What are the consequences? Lessons from the Dutch famine. Maturitas, 70(2), 141–145. https://doi.org/10.1016/j.maturitas.2011.06.017

Steinthorsdottir, V., Thorleifsson, G., Sulem, P., Helgason, H., Grarup, N., Sigurdsson, A., Helgadottir, H. T., Johannsdottir, H., Magnusson, O. T., Gudjonsson, S. A., Justesen, J. M., Harder, M. N., Jørgensen, M. E., Christensen, C., Brandslund, I., Sandbæk, A., Lauritzen, T., Vestergaard, H., Linneberg, A., … Stefansson, K. (2014). Identification of low-frequency and rare sequence variants associated with elevated or reduced risk of type 2 diabetes. Nature Genetics, 46(3), 294–298. https://doi.org/10.1038/ng.2882

Yajnik, C. S., Fall, C. H. D., Coyaji, K. J., Hirve, S. S., Rao, S., Barker, D. J. P., Joglekar, C., & Kellingray, S. (2003). Neonatal anthropometry: The thin–fat Indian baby. The Pune Maternal Nutrition Study. International Journal of Obesity, 27(2), Article 2. https://doi.org/10.1038/sj.ijo.802219

Yajnik, C. S., Lubree, H. G., Rege, S. S., Naik, S. S., Deshpande, J. A., Deshpande, S. S., Joglekar, C. V., & Yudkin, J. S. (2002). Adiposity and Hyperinsulinemia in Indians Are Present at Birth. The Journal of Clinical Endocrinology & Metabolism, 87(12), 5575–5580. https://doi.org/10.1210/jc.2002-020434

Chapter 3
Hey Doc, What is my Risk of a Heart Attack?

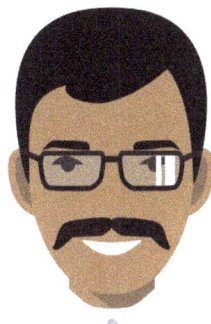

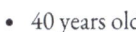
Rajinder

- Engineer in Toronto, Ontario
- Work is mostly sedentary (6-8 hours per day using a computer)
- Commute to work is 45mins one way
- Vegetarian
- Weight: 165lbs (up 20lbs since moving to Canada)
- Maternal family history of type 2 diabetes
- Father died of heart attack at age 60
- High Cholesterol
- Elevated Lipoprotein A

- 40 years old
- Overweight (BMI =26)
- Had gestational diabetes during her last pregnancy (at 30 years old)
- HBA1C of 5.9%
- Family history of diabetes and heart attacks
- Leads a sedentary lifestyle but is busy with 3 children
- Consumes a diet high in carbohydrates

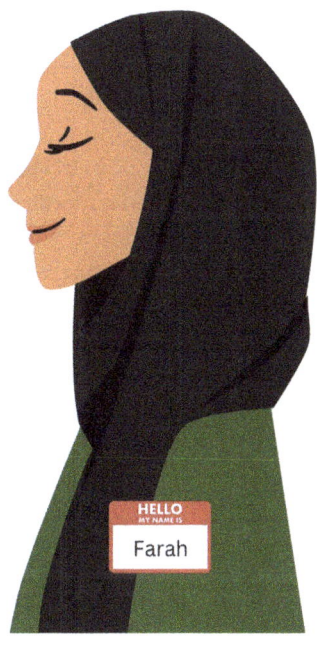
Farah

Everyone has a theory to explain why a loved one or friend suffered a sudden unexpected heart attack, often citing stress or a recent change in food intake. In this Chapter, I will focus on summarizing the scientific literature combined with my experience from treating patients in my clinic to show how risk for diabetes and heart attack is assessed. Let's start with a typical case:

Rajinder is a 40-year-old South Asian man who is referred to me because he is found to have "high cholesterol" identified on a workplace wellness assessment. He is otherwise well as indicated by his family doctor's note to me. I take his history in my clinic. He moved to Canada at age 20 years to do his master's degree and now works as an engineer in Toronto. His job is mostly sedentary- sitting at a computer for 6 of 8 hours per day plus his commute to work is 45 minutes by car each way. He is married and has two small children. He is asymptomatic from a cardiovascular standpoint, and exercises by playing racquetball with a friend twice per week. Since coming to Canada his weight has increased from 145 pounds on his 5'8" frame to 165 pounds - a change in his BMI from 22 to 25. When I asked him about his waist size change, he isn't really able to quantify this very well, his wife buys his clothes. He does comment that his brother from India tells him his face looks a little chubby. On further questioning about his family history, Rajinder tells you that his mother is alive at 65 years and has diabetes, but his father passed away suddenly of a suspected heart attack about 5 years ago at the age of 60 years. His only sibling - his brother is 45 years old and has no health issues. I asked him about his dietary intake. His food consumption is not excessive he reports. He is vegetarian. Breakfast is simple, lunch is something at the office – salad or soup, and he takes granola bars for snacks during the day. In the evening around 7 pm he has his evening meal – traditional Indian food, including chapati, daal, subzi, sometimes rice, and yogurt. He does not have dessert regularly but sometimes has some ice-cream later in the evening. He tries to avoid fast food – occasionally with the kids they order pizza, and on the weekend while socializing with other families he may have a larger Indian meal at another friend's home. He drinks a moderate amount of alcohol, either beer or scotch on the weekends. His physical exam reveals normal blood pressure, no identifiable signs of cardiovascular disease, but his waist circumference is elevated at 100 cm (39 inches), his BMI is 25, and his percent body fat is 40%. Review of his blood work shows that his non-HDL cholesterol is high at 4.66 mmol/L. His marker of long-term blood sugar HbA1C is borderline high at 5.9%, and his lipoprotein (a) is elevated at 80 mg/dL (172 nmol/L).

What should you do?

This story is typical amongst South Asian patients whom I see - usually they feel fine, and they have gone about their work and family life in a predictable manner and by their early 30s to middle age at 45 years of age, they have a blood test either for work insurance or for another health reason which reveals that they have elevated cholesterol or unexpectedly elevated blood sugar. This is not surprising if you are aware of the propensity of South Asians to gain weight like every other population group in **high** income or **urban** countries, where gaining 1 pound per year is not significantly noticed. Although among South Asians it is often around the middle, and arms and legs appear thin. **Cumulatively over the course of 20 years, this additional 20 pounds of weight gain can make a huge difference and impact on blood tests like cholesterol and blood sugar, especially so in South Asians.** Why is this? Well, this comes back to the thin fat phenotype and the fact that for every pound gained by a South Asian, is associated with more body fat per kilogram of body weight then observed in other ethnic groups. Thus, South Asians may look small stature typically based on height and the fact that fat stores are hidden around the waist and not that noticeable depending on the clothing worn. Among South Asian women this fat around the waist also translates into other ectopic regions including breast size. (Ray et al., 2008) Fat outside normal areas of storage include around the abdominal viscera, the liver, and around the heart - known as ectopic adipose tissue. Excess adiposity sets in motion a series of metabolic disruptions that can include changes in cholesterol, blood sugar, inflammatory markers, and signal that these abnormalities in metabolism are contributing to adverse health consequences. Wouldn't it be good to know this in advance of weight gain, wouldn't it be good to know that this happens in greater frequency among South Asians?

These questions led me and other researchers to try and determine when in the life course do these risk factors become apparent and in fact even before a baby is born, a mother's metabolic health influences her offspring's health. Thus, tips for expectant pregnant mothers who are South Asian include: trying to maintain a normal body weight, stay physically active, and hopefully be metabolically normal during pregnancy. South Asian expectant mothers should be tested for gestational glucose intolerance with a 75-gram oral glucose tolerance test. If gestational diabetes is found, this require a physician's guidance as how to manage it in pregnancy, and it is a marker that the mom has a two to threefold increase in developing type 2 diabetes in the next 10 to 15 years after delivery, as well as an increased risk of heart disease, and that her offspring is at risk for developing early onset type 2 diabetes.

Our research has shown that children start to develop evidence of metabolic abnormalities including elevated glucose at age 10 to 12 years and this is a precursor to developing early-onset type 2 diabetes. This process thus begins before birth and has been influenced by the offspring's parental genetics and the offspring's lifestyle and environment after birth. Recently, we showed that specific maternal and early life factors can lead to more or less fat tissue by age 3 years (Azab et al., 2025). Risks include high pre-pregnancy weight, weight gain during pregnancy, and screen time. Protective factors include breastfeeding, healthy diet during pregnancy, and physical activity. Knowing if there is a family history of diabetes and/or if the mother had gestational diabetes, parents can try to shape the newborns home environment to lower the risk of childhood overweight and obesity but **promoting healthy active living and minimizing sweets, junk food, soda pop, and screen time**. These are the ways in which South Asian children can grow up and prevent the early development of CV risk factors.

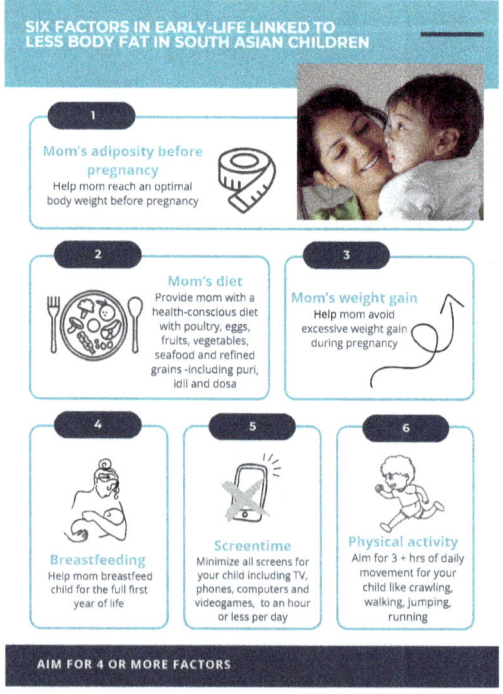

Measures of Blood sugar to detect pre-diabetes or diabetes: Our patient had a mildly elevated hemoglobin A1C (HbA1C) of 5.9%, what does this mean? Hemoglobin is a protein that is required by red blood cells to carry oxygen that is taken to our cell, tissues, and organs. When there are elevated levels of glucose circulating in the blood, glucose molecules bind to the hemoglobin protein. If these levels have been elevated for a prolonged period e.g. months this is reflected in an elevated HbA1c. Please see Table 1 below for ranges.

HbA1c%	
< 5.5%	Normal glucose metabolism
5.5-5.9%	Mild elevation of glucose
>/=6.0%	Likely glucose levels consistent with diabetes

Table 1: HbA1c% ranges

There are other methods of assessing diabetes and combinations of these measures, including measurement of fasting blood glucose, and post glucose 75-gram load glucose levels. The advantage of the HbA1c is it gives a fairly accurate picture of the last three months and is not assessing recent dietary or fasting state. Most physicians use this marker in clinical practice as well. If your HbA1C is normal < 5.5%, the sensitivity to rule out diabetes is high (Ekoe et al., 2018). If it is elevated, >/6.5% the specificity is very high, and may lead your doctor to repeat this together with a fasting and or 2-hour glucose to confirm the diagnosis of diabetes (Ekoe et al., 2018).

There are some risk calculators for type 2 diabetes available. In Figure 1 the risk calculator developed in South India shows you the key variables (minus genetic factors) that are associated with risk. A high score is closely correlated with elevated blood sugar which is used to diagnose type 2 diabetes.

However, in high income countries, it is not difficult nor costly for most people to have their blood sugar checked via primary care specialists. Thus, it is very reasonable to measure one's blood sugar with regular blood work and certainly important to do this more frequently amongst individuals with risk factors such as strong family history, abdominal obesity, age of 50 years, and those who live a very sedentary lifestyle. Patients are often surprised when their routine bloodwork shows an elevated blood sugar but given all that you know now it should not be that surprising. The path to cardio-metabolic risk unfortunately starts very early in life among South Asians.

Risk Factor	Score
Age	
35 years	0
35-49 years	20
≥ 50 years	30
Abdominal Obesity	
Waist circumference Female <80 cm or Male <90 cm (Reference)	0
Female 80-89 cm or Male 90-99 cm	10
Female ≥ 90 cm or Male ≥ 100 cm	20
Physical Activity	
Vigorous exercise or strenuous at work	0
Exercise at work/home	10
Mild exercise at work/home	20
No exercise and sedentary at work/home	30
Family History	
Two non-diabetic parents	0
Either parent diabetic	10
Both parents diabetic	20
Your score	
Maximum score	100
Key ≥ 60: High risk 30-50: Medium risk < 30: Low risk	
Your risk category	

Table 2: Madras Diabetes Research Foundation Indian Diabetes Risk Score (MDRF IDRS) (Mohan et al., 2005).

Cholesterol Profile: Receiving a cholesterol measurement from your doctor can be confusing – because there are so many values to consider and that can be used.

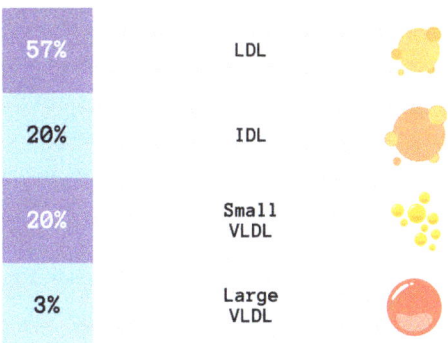

Figure 2: Schematic of the various LDL subclasses along with their recommended assays (Adapted from Holmes & Ala-Korpela, 2019).

The common metrics used include "bad" or LDL cholesterol, "good" or HDL cholesterol, triglycerides, or some combinations or ratios of these. As the picture depicts, there are bad or atherogenic lipoproteins which increase the amount of "sludge in your pipes" or atherosclerosis in your arteries. Some components of your cholesterol profile like high HDL cholesterol are markers of a lower risk person. After many decades of research clinical practice guidelines recommend targets that focus on "LDL" cholesterol, or non-HDL cholesterol, fasting or non-fasting. The parameters used by different countries reflect a few factors - tradition, laboratory measurements, costs, and national guidelines. That is why there is variation between countries, and even within countries, on what is measured and what advise stems from these.

To simplify, the Table 2 indicates for "Primary Prevention" like our patient case what is considered high or abnormal.

Lipid Measure	Fasting (mmol/L)	Non-Fasting mmol/L
Total Cholesterol mmol/L	< 5.2	< 5.2
LDL Cholesterol mmol/L	< 3.50	Not accurate
HDL Cholesterol mmol/L	>1.00	>1.00
Non-HDL Cholesterol (Total cholesterol minus HDL cholesterol) mmol/L	<2.66	<2.66
Triglycerides mmol/L	< 2.26	Not accurate

Table 2: Lipid measures

For individuals who have already suffered a heart attack, or some clinical manifestation of vascular disease this is called "Secondary Prevention", and all guidelines recommend cholesterol lowering medications most notably STATINS, and although different guidelines and countries indicate different targets, a general rule of thumb is for every 1 mmol/L reduction in LDL cholesterol equates to a 20% reduction in recurrent cardiovascular events – so in short **"lower is better"**.

In the Chapter 7 on medical therapies, you will find the usual approach to selection of cholesterol agents in both primary and secondary prevention.

Other Lipid or Fat Biomarkers in your Blood that can point to genetic risk:

Lipoprotein (a): This lipoprotein is a fascinating suspect in the mystery of early onset and sometimes fatal myocardial infraction. As you can see in the picture below it is an awkward Lipoprotein that has attached to it multiple small molecules called crinkle for repeats. It is 90% genetically mediated and therefore runs in families. Lp(a) can be implicated in sudden death or unexpected early onset heart attacks. It is a apolipoprotein that is associated with creating more "sludge in the pipes" referring arteries, as well as forming blood clots through complex mechanisms related to the KIV repeats.

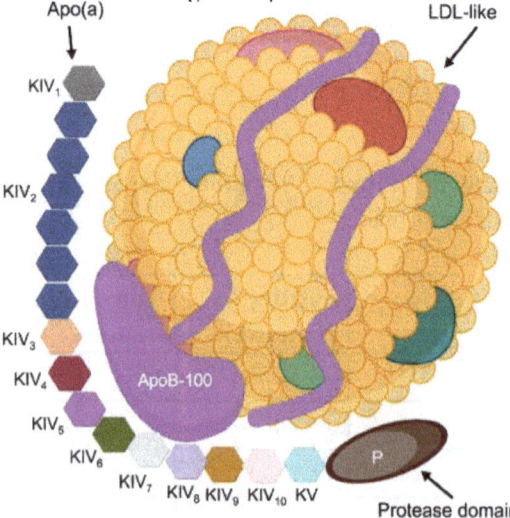

Figure 3: Structure of Lipoprotein (a) which is composed of two main parts: LDL-like particles and apolipoprotein (a). (Reprinted from Liu et al., 2021).

This factor is a complicated yet fascinating story to tell. The high circulating levels of this lipid-protein can lead to more atherosclerosis or "sludge in the arteries" and blood clotting. Amongst South Asians who you hear "had no risk factors" yet suffered a devastating heart attack, elevated levels of Lp(a) might be the cause (Anand et al., 1998). There is a strong genetic link with Lp(a) – it runs in families. South Asians grouped together have a higher mean level than do other ethnic groups, and it is a risk factor for heart attack (Paré et al., 2019).

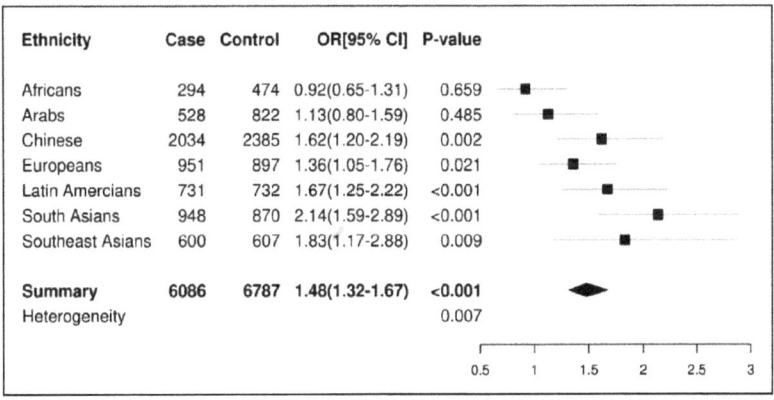

Figure 4: Association of high lipoprotein(a) [Lp(a)] concentrations (>50 mg/dL) with myocardial infarction for each ethnic group. (Reprinted from Paré et al., 2019).

It is 90% genetically mediated and autosomal dominant, therefore if your level comes back high, one of your parents also had this elevated blood lipid-protein. It is advisable to have this value checked at least once in your lifetime because it is genetically transmitted. Repeating this measure over time is not advised unless advised by your doctor.

There are interesting hypotheses as to the evolutionary advantage of having high Lp(a) explaining why it persists in the population. High Lp(a) is observed in equator-dwelling populations – suggesting that high Lp(a) has a protective effect against certain infections like malaria or other bacterial infections. There are other hypotheses that it is an efficient cholesterol transporter and therefore can heal an injured artery, however in modern times, with higher cholesterol this accelerated transportation leads to early atherosclerosis. It has also been proposed that the physiological role of Lp(a) may be to promote wound healing. Lp(a) is conformationally similar to a protein involved in blood clotting called plasminogen – and because of this may prevent the conversion of plasminogen to plasmin – plasmin is like circulating "draino" mopping up clotting factors and breaking down tiny blood clots – without this efficient housekeeper blood clots may be more likely to form. Even the lowly hedgehog has an elevated Lp(a) to protect it from bleeding to death from the advances of venomous snakes.

How is high Lipoprotein (a) treated?

There are not many treatments for high Lp(a), and we still don't know if reducing the level in the blood stream reduces the risk of recurrent cardiovascular disease. An RNA anti sense molecule is being tested now in clinical trials to determine if lowering Lp(a) production lowers clinical risk of CVD. Pelacarsen is an antisense oligonucleotide AKCEA-APO(a)-LRx which effectively reduces Lp(a) levels by up to 80% by impairing the synthesis of apolipoprotein(a) (Tsimikas et al., 2020). Other Lp(a) disrupters include drugs called Olpasiran and Zerlasiran – all of which are currently in clinical trial testing. These studies are underway, so it is too soon to know if they will be effective in lowering not only lipoprotein (a) but also clinical events. For now, to prevent heart attacks and strokes – we recommend the cholesterol level is lowered by use of medications such as statins, with add-on ezetimibe, and in some cases PCSK-9 inhibitors. Sometimes individuals with elevated Lp(a) and a history of blood clotting are also placed on blood thinning agents including aspirin plus or minus a more potent blood thinner.

How do I know if I have high Lipoprotein (a)?

You can speak with your primary care doctor or specialist and request this test to be checked. There is lab to lab variation in the assay used to measure Lp(a) – but very high levels are usually indicative that you "have the risk factor". The Canadian Cardiovascular Society lipid guidelines recommend that "all people have Lp(a) measured at least once in their lifetime" to help risk stratify for future CVD. They go on to recommend earlier and more intensive behaviour modification and ASCVD risk factor management is recommended for those with a Lp(a) ≥50 mg/dL (or ≥100 nmol/L) (Pearson et al., 2021).

Bringing it back to the patient:
Our patient Rajinder, at the beginning of this chapter, had a number of issues, he had excess adipose tissue [increased waist circumference, BMI, percent body fat – all three of these measures pointed that out!]; increased

non-HDL cholesterol, increased Lp(a) and mildly elevated HbA1c. On the good side, his blood pressure was normal and he didn't smoke. Using our INTERHEART Risk Score (see Appendix 1 for lab-based risk score)– Rajinder would be classified as low to moderate risk of a future heart attack. A large study of apparently health people we conducted in Canada, in which all participants underwent magnetic resonance imaging scans to search for early sign of vascular disease showed that the percent with vascular disease already apparent in the arteries in the low, moderate, and high risk groups were 30%, 50% and 65% for men. That means that with this set of risk factors: excess adiposity, abnormal cholesterol, high Lp(a), and pre diabetes, the probability that Rajinder has pre-clinical atherosclerosis, the precursor to heart attacks and stroke is quite high. Even though he can't "feel" it, he needs to quickly move toward risk factor normalization, to prevent a sudden, surprise of a heart attack, and full-blown type 2 diabetes.

	IHRS Low	IHRS Moderate	IHR High	Statistical Significance
Carotid wall volume (mm^3)	881.5 (163.1)	915.4 (166.6)	940.9 (172.9)	<0.0001
Intraplaque Hemorrhage	1.8%	3.0%	3.1%	0.001
MRI-detected cerebrovascular disease	4.5	7.5%	8.9%	<0.001

Table 3: Percent with subclinical atherosclerosis or carotid, intraplaque hemorrhage, or vascular brain injury detected by MRI (Anand et al., 2019)

For Rajinder, at his first clinic visit, I would discuss fat loss strategies which includes dietary and activity changes namely: carbohydrate reduction by 50% (see SAHARA diet chart, and section 2,3,4), regular physical activity, and initiation of a statin medication. I would propose re-measuring his blood tests including HbA1C in 3 months; and add to his bloodwork liver enzymes. I sent him home with a dietary brochure, and describe that although I am starting one medication today and have provided a lot of advice to him – the long game for doing this is to prevent a clinical cardiovascular event – even though he is reluctant to take medication; I emphasized that if he suffered a heart attack, he would leave hospital on no fewer than 4 medications. This is usually a motivating factor for most patients to start their medication for cholesterol or blood pressure lowering as prescribed.

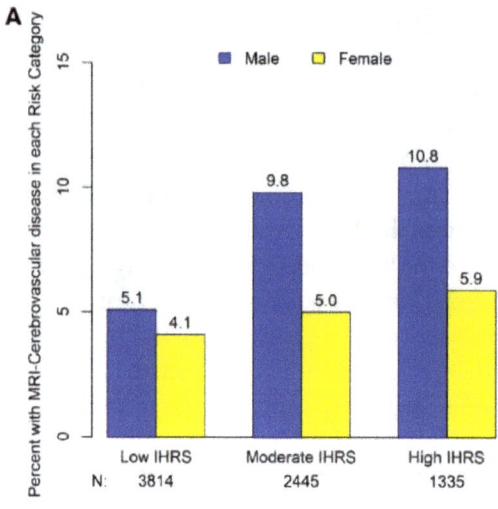

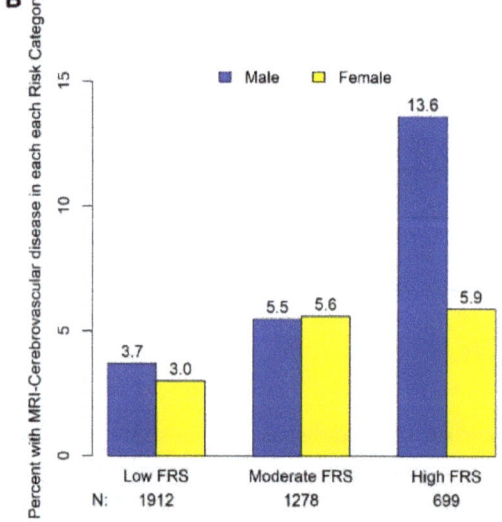

Figure 5: (A) Proportion of cohort with combined MRI-detected cerebrovascular disease within INTERHEART risk score (IHRS) category by sex. (B) Proportion of cohort with combined MRI-detected cerebrovascular disease within Framingham Risk Score (FRS) category by sex (Reprinted from Anand et al., 2019).

Case 2: Gestational diabetes - an early warning sign for women regarding their future risk of diabetes and cardiovascular disease.

Farah is age 40 years. She was born in Pakistan and came to Canada when she was 4 years old. Her BMI is 26 (this is overweight) and she had gestational diabetes mellitus (GDM) during her last pregnancy at age 30 years. This was discovered on oral glucose tolerance testing. Farah prompted her primary care doctor to make the referral to me because her blood work now shows a HbA1C of 5.9%, her history of GDM, along with her family history as her father and mother both have type 2 diabetes, and her father had his first heart attack at age 60 year. Her family doctor having recently attended a conference learned that GDM is a risk factor for cardiovascular disease in women, now sends her to you – the CV specialist to seek medical advice regarding her future risk of cardiovascular disease (CVD) after experiencing gestational diabetes.

Your more detailed history reveals that Farah was diagnosed with GDM during her second trimester of her third pregnancy. She managed her condition through dietary modifications and regular exercise, successfully controlling her blood glucose levels. You inquire about her weight at the time she was married (at age 20 years) which she reports was 122 pounds (55 kilograms), and for a person 5'4" or 162.6 cm, her BMI was 21. Piecing together her history, she reports that with each pregnancy she never was able to return to her pre-pregnancy weight as life got busy, she had little time for exercise, and often found herself finishing her children's plate of leftovers. All this change in lifestyle, along with 2 pregnancies, has resulted in her weight gain of 30 pounds over ten years!

Farah is married and lives with her husband and three young children. She leads a sedentary lifestyle given the demands of young motherhood and her office job. She follows a predominantly South Asian diet, which includes high-carbohydrate intake made up of rice and roti, and when at work she buys a sandwich. On weekends she and her husband both exhausted from their busy weeks, typically pack up their three kids and head out for pizza or other restaurant style foods.

Apart from her weight gain, you measure her waist circumference and measure that she is above the waist circumference target for a South Asian woman (Normal </=80 cm). Farah's waist measures 95 cm. Luckily her blood pressure and cholesterol remain in the normal range, but her

HbA1C is 5.9%, which is in the "pre-diabetes" range.

Plan: Unfortunately, Farah's current state of weight gain/retention over successive pregnancies is common. Among South Asian women the fat distribution is usual central. The fact that she was diagnosed with gestational diabetes increases her risk of developing diabetes by 2-3 times.

In our 2021 paper we summarized the risks of GDM for pregnant women and their offspring Women diagnosed with GDM, compared to those without, have a **seven-fold higher lifetime risk of T2DM**, and 50% of them develop T2DM within five years of giving birth (Desai et al., 2021). GDM predicts future vascular disease in the mother, and increases the risk of T2DM **in her offspring up to eight times** (Desai et al., 2021). South Asian women have **double the risk of GDM** of white European women, and therefore may not be aware of their risk from regular health care they receive in North America (Desai et al., 2021). Their offspring also have increased risk factors for future T2DM, including higher birth weight, more adipose tissue, and reduced insulin sensitivity (Desai et al., 2021). These risk factors are appreciably more common in South Asian infants born to mothers with GDM than infants born to mothers without GDM (Anand et al., 2017).

In our previous studies we have shown that 36% of South Asian women in Ontario, Canada develop GDM (Desai et al., 2021). Furthermore, a poor-quality diet during pregnancy increases the chances of developing GDM (odds ratio [OR]: 1.62; 95% CI: 1.20 to 2.19) (Desai et al., 2021). Poor diet quality is high in ultra-processed foods, sweets, rice, and fast foods. Indeed, our finding that ≈13% of GDM cases in this population could be prevented if diet quality were improved, highlights the value of high diet quality to prevent GDM (Desai et al., 2021). Our research suggests that improving diet quality in the Canadian population of South Asian pregnant women may therefore prevent up to 6500 new T2DM cases by 2031 (Desai et al., 2021).

The role of physical activity will be discussed in more depth in Chapter 5. Without question, regular physical activity which increases one's heart rate and breathing is associated with significant overall health benefits. In the case of preventing GDM, the strongest modifiable risk factors for South Asians appear to be a woman's pre-pregnancy weight and diet quality. Thus, the preparation of South Asian women planning for pregnancy

includes diet and activity counselling - ideally before pregnancy.
In the SMART Start study we created a multi-media toolkit consisting of an informational video narrative, illustrated booklet, and summary material created to attempt to change knowledge, attitudes, practices, and confidence in making healthy active living changes among South Asian women in pregnancy (Kandasamy et al., 2024).

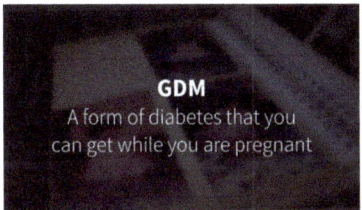
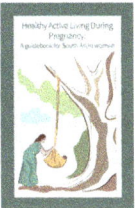
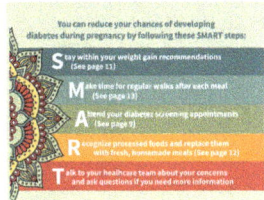

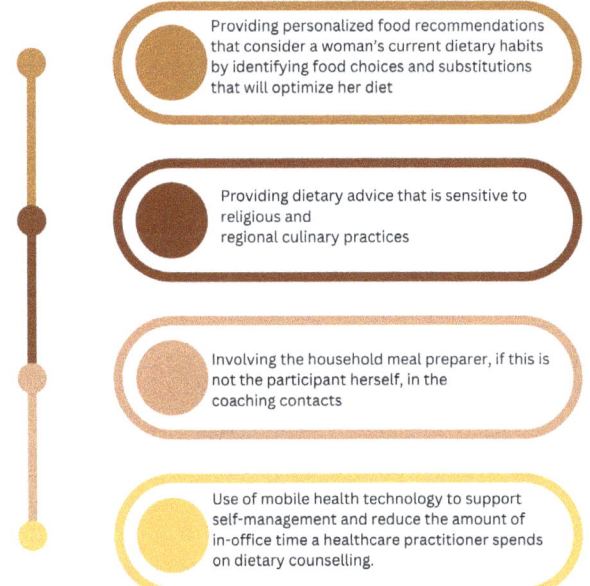

DESI-GDM
DIETARY PRINCIPLES

 Replacing traditional fried foods and meat with more vegetable protein and raw and cooked vegetables

Reducing carbohydrate intake, for those who report consumption of high quantities of refined carbohydrates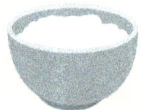

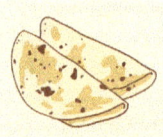 Improving carbohydrate quality (replacing high glycaemic index, refined-grain foods with lower glycaemic index, whole-grain foods (e.g., replacing white rice with parboiled rice, brown rice, or legumes; replacing white flour paratha with whole wheat paratha)

Reducing trans fats (e.g., switching from commercial ghee to butter or vegetable oil)

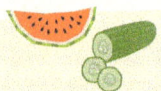 Scheduling regular mealtimes, 3–4 h apart

Replacing fried, high-carbohydrate snacks (e.g., chaat or dahi vada) with higher protein and fat snacks (such as nuts or full-fat dairy)

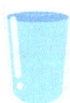 Replacing sweets and sugar-sweetened drinks (sweetened chai, soda pop, and juice) with water or unsweetened tea and choosing fruits and other lower-sugar desserts over desserts high in starch and sugar

In this program we found that healthy active living is a topic area with a high degree of interest among South Asian pregnant women and their family physicians; specifically, that pregnant patients valued the new prenatal information they learned, improved some of their physical activity and dietary behaviours, and made recommendations for improving future prenatal health communication (Kandasamy et al., 2024). However, we also observed that even though knowledge was valued by patients and their doctors, it was very difficult for pregnant women to make changes in their eating and exercising patterns on their own. This demonstrates that **social support and group motivation to encourage and reinforce healthy dietary changes** is a crucial piece to the puzzle. Many of these principles of behavioural support have been shown to be effective in other settings and programs such as the Weight Watchers model which offers support through meetings, online communities, and personalized coaching, creating a sense of accountability and encouragement (Tate et al., 2022).

Our prescription for pregnant South Asian women to prevent GDM is informed by a series of studies we conducted in Canada, and are currently testing this "recipe" in a randomized clinical trial (Stennett, 2023).

In Farah's case, she was being assessed 10 years after she finished having children. Advice for her now includes consuming a balanced high quality foods diet, regular exercise, and weight management, as the mainstay of her management.

Cardiovascular Risk Assessment: Given Farah's history of GDM, combined with her family history of diabetes and high blood pressure, she has an increased risk of developing cardiovascular disease.

A comprehensive cardiovascular risk assessment was conducted, including evaluating her lipid profile, blood pressure, and body fat. This assessment helped to determine her individual risk factors and guide targeted interventions.

1. **Lifestyle Modifications**: Farah will receive counseling regarding the importance of maintaining a healthy lifestyle. She will be encouraged to adopt a balanced diet, rich in fruits, vegetables, whole grains, lean proteins, and healthy fats, while minimizing processed foods, sugary beverages, and saturated fats. Regular physical activity, such as brisk walking or moderate-intensity exercise, will be encouraged to improve insulin sensitivity and overall cardiovascular health.

2. **Regular Follow-up**: Farah will be scheduled for regular follow-up visits to monitor her glycemic control, lipid profile, blood pressure, and weight. These visits will provide an opportunity to assess her adherence to lifestyle modifications, address any concerns or challenges, and make necessary adjustments to her treatment plan.
3. **Long-Term Cardiovascular Monitoring**: Farah's cardiovascular health will be closely monitored over the years to assess her risk of developing CVD. This will involve periodic lipid profile assessments, blood pressure checks, and counseling on managing other modifiable risk factors, such as smoking cessation and stress reduction.
4. **Patient Education**: Farah will receive comprehensive education regarding the relationship between GDM and future cardiovascular risk. She will be empowered with knowledge about the importance of early intervention, long-term monitoring, and sustained lifestyle modifications to reduce her risk of CVD.
5. **Monitoring her blood glucose periodically** will help detect any early signs of dysglycemia, and if her HbA1C increases into the diabetic range she will need medication (see Chapter 7).
6. **Farah will also be informed of the increased her GDM places upon her three growing children**, their risk of developing earlier onset diabetes and resources to create an environment where high quality foods and ample physical activity through sports and other physical activity is the norm.

By implementing lifestyle modifications and close follow-up, both Rajinder and Farah could reduce their future risk of diabetes, metabolic syndrome, and cardiovascular disease.

How does risk change with age? Aging is the strongest risk factors for risk of heart disease, and therefore the absolute risk increase of heart disease increases every decade. However, there are certain stages in the life course that change the risk trajectory significantly. Most notable among women, pregnancy, and after menopause (average age of 50 years) are stages in the life course where some risk factors become apparent. In Farah's case she had pregnancy related GDM, other women have high blood pressure in pregnancy – both provide insight into the women's future risk of heart and vascular disease being higher than for women without these risk factors. Women were traditionally thought to the "protected" from heart disease until regular menstrual periods stopped with aging. In menopause, where endogenous estrogen levels are lower, women bodies change, and they are more likely to develop central or visceral adiposity, and associated increase in cholesterol, blood pressure, and blood sugar, such that by age 60 years women and men's physiology is quite similar. For males, smoking is more common, and this is a strong risk factor for heart disease, stroke, and peripheral artery disease. Males also have more visceral adiposity than females, and if this occurs early in life e.g. before the age of 30 years then other cardiometabolic risk factors may also develop earlier than average. Finally, globally obesity is on the risk and obesity is a risk factor to women and men, and sadly is becoming more common in childhood. Obesity shortens the lifespan of men and women, such that today's children with obesity are not expected to outlive their parents. (Figure 6)

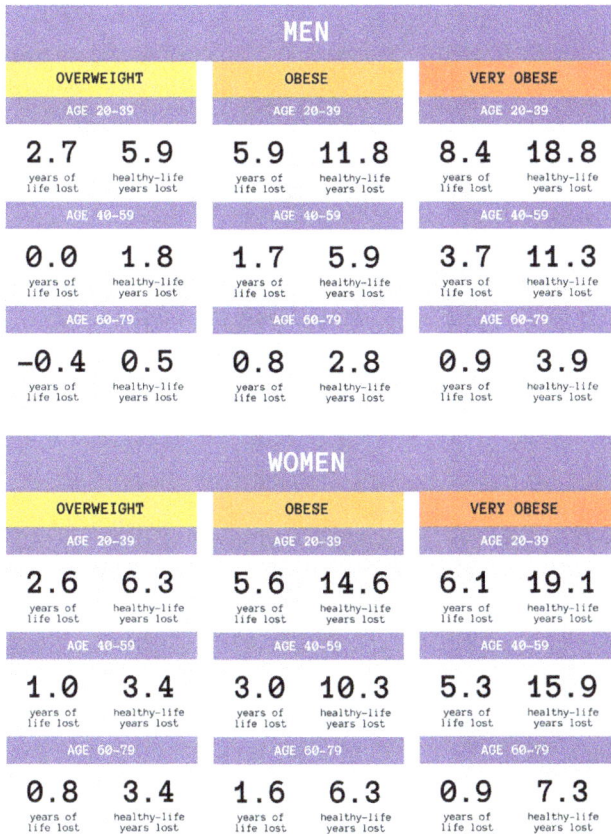

Figure 6: Comparison of years of life lost and healthy-life years lost in men and women, compared to those with an ideal body weight (Adapted from Grover et al., 2015).

REFERENCES

Anand, S. S., Enas, E. A., Pogue, J., Haffner, S., Pearson, T., & Yusuf, S. (1998). Elevated lipoprotein(a) levels in South Asians in North America. Metabolism: Clinical and Experimental, 47(2), 182–184. https://doi.org/10.1016/s0026-0495(98)90217-7

Anand, S. S., Gupta, M., Teo, K. K., Schulze, K. M., Desai, D., Abdalla, N., Zulyniak, M., de Souza, R., Wahi, G., Shaikh, M., Beyene, J., de Villa, E., Morrison, K., McDonald, S. D., & Gerstein, H. (2017). Causes and consequences of gestational diabetes in South Asians living in Canada: Results from a prospective cohort study. CMAJ Open, 5(3), E604–E611. https://doi.org/10.9778/cmajo.20170027

Anand, S. S., Tu, J. V., Desai, D., Awadalla, P., Robson, P., Jacquemont, S., Dummer, T., Le, N., Parker, L., Poirier, P., Teo, K., Lear, S. A., Yusuf, S., Tardif, J.-C., Marcotte, F., Busseuil, D., Després, J.-P., Black, S. E., Kirpalani, A., ... on behalf of the Canadian Alliance for Healthy Hearts and Minds Cohort. (2019). Cardiovascular risk scoring and magnetic resonance imaging detected subclinical cerebrovascular disease. European Heart Journal - Cardiovascular Imaging, 21(6), 692–700. https://doi.org/10.1093/ehjci/jez226

Azab, S. M., Naqvi, S., Rafiq, T., Beyene, J., Deng, W., Lamri, A., ... & Anand, S. S. (2025). Trajectory of Early Life Adiposity Among South Asian Children. JAMA Network Open, 8(4), e254439-e254439

Desai, D., Kandasamy, S., Limbachia, J., Zulyniak, M. A., Ritvo, P., Sherifali, D., Wahi, G., Anand, S. S., & de Souza, R. J. (2021). Studies to Improve Perinatal Health through Diet and Lifestyle among South Asian Women Living in Canada: A Brief History and Future Research Directions. Nutrients, 13(9), Article 9. https://doi.org/10.3390/nu13092932

Ekoe, J.-M., Goldenberg, R., & Katz, P. (2018). Screening for Diabetes in Adults. Canadian Journal of Diabetes, 42, S16–S19. https://doi.org/10.1016/j.jcjd.2017.10.004

Grover, S. A., Kaouache, M., Rempel, P., Joseph, L., Dawes, M., Lau, D. C. W., & Lowensteyn, I. (2015). Years of life lost and healthy life-years lost from diabetes and cardiovascular disease in overweight and obese people: A modelling study. The Lancet. Diabetes & Endocrinology, 3(2), 114–122. https://doi.org/10.1016/S2213-8587(14)70229-3

Holmes, M. V., & Ala-Korpela, M. (2019). What is 'LDL cholesterol'? Nature Reviews Cardiology, 16(4), Article 4. https://doi.org/10.1038/s41569-019-0157-6

Kandasamy, S., Amjad, S., de Souza, R., Furqan, N., Patel, T., Vanstone, M., & Anand, S. S. (2024). Getting a "SMART START" to gestational diabetes mellitus education: A mixed-methods pilot evaluation of a knowledge translation tool in primary care. Family Practice, cmad119. https://doi.org/10.1093/fampra/cmad119

Liu, T., Yoon, W.-S., & Lee, S.-R. (2021). Recent Updates of Lipoprotein(a) and Cardiovascular Disease. Chonnam Medical Journal, 57(1), 36–43. https://doi.org/10.4068/cmj.2021.57.1.36

Mohan, V., Deepa, R., Deepa, M., Somannavar, S., & Datta, M. (2005). A simplified Indian Diabetes Risk Score for screening for undiagnosed diabetic subjects. The Journal of the Association of Physicians of India, 53, 759–763.

Paré, G., Çaku, A., McQueen, M., Anand, S. S., Enas, E., Clarke, R., Boffa, M. B., Koschinsky, M., Wang, X., Yusuf, S., & null, null. (2019). Lipoprotein(a) Levels and the Risk of Myocardial Infarction Among 7 Ethnic Groups. Circulation, 139(12), 1472–1482. https://doi.org/10.1161/CIRCULATIONAHA.118.034311

Pearson, G. J., Thanassoulis, G., Anderson, T. J., Barry, A. R., Couture, P., Dayan, N., Francis, G. A., Genest, J., Grégoire, J., Grover, S. A., Gupta, M., Hegele, R. A., Lau, D., Leiter, L. A., Leung, A. A., Lonn, E., Mancini, G. B. J., Manjoo, P., McPherson, R., … Wray, W. (2021). 2021 Canadian Cardiovascular Society Guidelines for the Management of Dyslipidemia for the Prevention of Cardiovascular Disease in Adults. Canadian Journal of Cardiology, 37(8), 1129–1150. https://doi.org/10.1016/j.cjca.2021.03.016

Ray, J. G., Mohllajee, A. P., Dam, R. M. van, & Michels, K. B. (2008). Breast size and risk of type 2 diabetes mellitus. CMAJ, 178(3), 289–295. https://doi.org/10.1503/cmaj.071086

Stennett, R. N., Adamo, K. B., Anand, S. S., Bajaj, H. S., Bangdiwala, S. I., Desai, D., … & de Souza, R. J. (2023). A culturally tailored personaliseD nutrition intErvention in South ASIan women at risk of Gestational Diabetes Mellitus (DESI-GDM): a randomised controlled trial protocol. BMJ open, 13(5), e072353.

Tate, D. F., Lutes, L. D., Bryant, M., Truesdale, K. P., Hatley, K. E., Griffiths, Z., Tang, T. S., Padgett, L. D., Pinto, A. M., Stevens, J., & Foster, G. D. (2022). Efficacy of a Commercial Weight Management Program Compared With a Do-It-Yourself Approach: A Randomized Clinical Trial. JAMA Network Open, 5(8), e2226561. https://doi.org/10.1001/jamanetworkopen.2022.26561

Tsimikas, S., Karwatowska-Prokopczuk, E., Gouni-Berthold, I., Tardif, J.-C., Baum, S. J., Steinhagen-Thiessen, E., Shapiro, M. D., Stroes, E. S., Moriarty, P. M., Nordestgaard, B. G., Xia, S., Guerriero, J., Viney, N. J., O'Dea, L., & Witztum, J. L. (2020). Lipoprotein(a) Reduction in Persons with Cardiovascular Disease. New England Journal of Medicine, 382(3), 244–255. https://doi.org/10.1056/NEJMoa1905239

APPENDIX A: INTERHEART RISK SCORE

Risk factor	Question	Points for the answer		Points for each section
Age	Are you a man 55 years or older OR woman 65 years or older?		2	Points:
	OR Are you a man younger than 55 years or woman younger than 65 years		0	
Smoking. Pick the description which matches you best:	I never smoked		0	Points:
	OR I am a former smoker (last smoked more than 12 months ago)		2	
	OR I am a current smoker or I smoked regularly in the last months, and I smoke…	1-5 cigarettes per day	2	
		6-10 cigarettes per 12 day	4	
		11-15 cigarettes per day	6	
		16-20 cigarettes per day	7	
		More than 20 cigarettes per day	11	
Second hand smoke	Over the past 12 months, what has been your typical exposure to other people's tobacco smoke	Less than 1 hour or exposure per week or no exposure	0	Points:
		OR One or more hours of secondhand smoke exposure per week	2	
Diabetes	Do you have diabetes mellitus?	Yes	6	Points:
		No or unsure	0	
High Blood Pressure	Do you have high blood pressure?	Yes	5	Points:
		No or unsure	0	
Family History	Have either or both of your biological parents had a heart attack?	Yes	4	Points:
		No or unsure	0	
Waist to hip ratio	Pick one only:	Quartile 1: Less than 0.873	0	Points:
		Quartile 2 & 3: 0.873 - 0.963	2	
		Quartile 4: Greater than or = 0.964	4	
Psychosocial factors	How often have you felt work or home life stress in the last year? Pick one only	Never or some periods	0	Points:
		OR Several periods of stress or permanent stress	3	

	During the past 12 months, was there ever a time when you felt sad, blue, or depressed for two weeks or more in a row?	Yes	3	**Points:**
		No	0	
Dietary factors. Pick one answer for each food group mentioned	Do you eat salty food or snacks one or more times a day	Yes	1	**Points:**
		No	0	
	Do you eat deep fried foods or snacks or fast foods 3 or more times a week?	Yes	1	**Points:**
		No	0	
	Do you eat fruit one or more times daily?	Yes	0	**Points:**
		No	1	
	Do you eat vegetables one or more times daily?	Yes	0	**Points:**
		No	1	
	Do you eat meat and/or poultry 2 or more times daily?	Yes	2	**Points:**
		No	0	
Physical activity	How active are you during your leisure time?	I am mainly sedentary or perform mild exercise (requiring minimal effort)	2	**Points:**
		OR I perform moderate or strenuous physical activity in my leisure time	0	

* In this table, the categories of the risk factors are presented in the first column, and the specific questions to be asked in the middle columns. Only one answer is chosen for every question, and inserted into the "points" column. All questions must be answered for the most accurate risk score estimate. The IHRS for an individual is calculated by adding the points from each of the above items.

Chapter 4
What role does diet play?

What role does diet play in the development of South Asian risk factors?

Most people have absorbed from the media, confusing dietary guidelines, and from their own doctors, that **all fat is bad** for them, and that **consumption of fatty foods** causes high cholesterol and then heart disease. But is this true? If it is true, then yes, we should be emphasizing to all South Asians to reduce all sources of fat consumption to prevent them from needing a cholesterol lowering pill and to prevent heart disease. However, you will see below those simple carbohydrates (e.g. white polished rice, bread, white pasta, most sugary desserts) may be the most deleterious for South Asians, and thus a lower carbohydrate balanced food consumption is advised.

Dietary Patterns and Cardio-metabolic Risk: From the perspective of foods, population studies show that there is a substantial proportion of South Asians particularly those of the Hindu religion, **who are vegetarian**. In our population-based studies in North America this percentage is about 18 to 20% of South Asians. Among vegetarians who do not consume meat products, carbohydrate consumption is usually higher to make up for these calories. The typical vegetarian South Asian dietary pattern includes substantial carbohydrate intake making up 60% of daily energy intake, usually in the form of traditional South Asian foods such as rice and roti. Carbohydrates made up of relatively higher amounts of sugar and lower fibre are linked to apple shaped fat distribution (Merchant et al., 2005).

Carbohydrates can be high in sugar and low in fiber, or they can be higher in fiber. So not all carbohydrates are bad, the carbohydrates to avoid based on current evidence are those that increase the glycemic index or have a high glycemic load, meaning the response to consuming such foods results in a rapid increase in glucose and insulin shortly after the food is consumed. **These foods typically are simple carbohydrates, this includes sugar, and processed carbohydrates including refined grains, such as white polished rice. It also includes the typical foods in North**

America such as white bread and desserts, and sugar sweetened beverages which are high in sugar. All of these foods will increase the glycemic index and load, and this has been associated with an increased risk are diabetes, central obesity known as the Canadian Tire, as well as death (de Koning et al., 2007, Jenkins et al., 2021).

Goal	Intervention
Prevention of weight gain	Eucaloric balanced diet
(Primary prevention)	30–60 min of moderate exercise
Obesity treatment	
– induction of weight loss	Hypocaloric diet
	60–120 min of moderate exercise
– weight loss maintenance	Calorie-restricted diet*
(Secondary prevention)	90–120 min of vigorous exercise

Table 1: Simple Tips to Manage Abdominal Obesity (Merchant et al., 2006)
*May require addition of anti-obesity medication or surgical intervention.

Quit sugary beverages: Soda pop consumption is common in certain communities, at parties or get togethers, as a thirst quencher. Most people don't think twice about having a can of ginger ale or coca cola. Unfortunately, there is a significant amount of sugar in soda pop, and regular consumption is associated with weight gain, type 2 diabetes, and death in adults, and weight gain and type 2 diabetes in children (Grimes et al., 2013; Imamura et al., 2016; Malik et al., 2010; Pan et al., 2014; Wang et al., 2015). Some countries have moved to curb the consumption of soda pop by imposing a tax of up to 20% on these drinks. The best option is to eliminate these drinks from your intake. If this is hard for you, consider replacing soda pop with diet versions that have low to no calories. There is some controversy about the impact of diet drinks on the gut microbiome and taste/hunger centre -but as this information is still inconclusive, it seems prudent to switch from non-diet version to diet versions as a first step.

How then in an urban lifestyle with the need to use convenience foods and consume foods out of restaurants or convenience snacks, can people who are predisposed to developing cardiometabolic disorders replace these foods with higher quality foods? The high-quality carbohydrates include those that are grain-based with a high fiber component, and a general rule of thumb which is reasonable to follow is, for every food the ratio of carbohydrates to fibre should be 10:1, if it is higher e.g. 20:1 then the food lacks enough fibre to slow absorption from the gut. For example, choose bread that for one slice has 8 grams of carbohydrate to 1 of fibre, rather than 20 grams of carbohydrate to 1 gram of fibre.

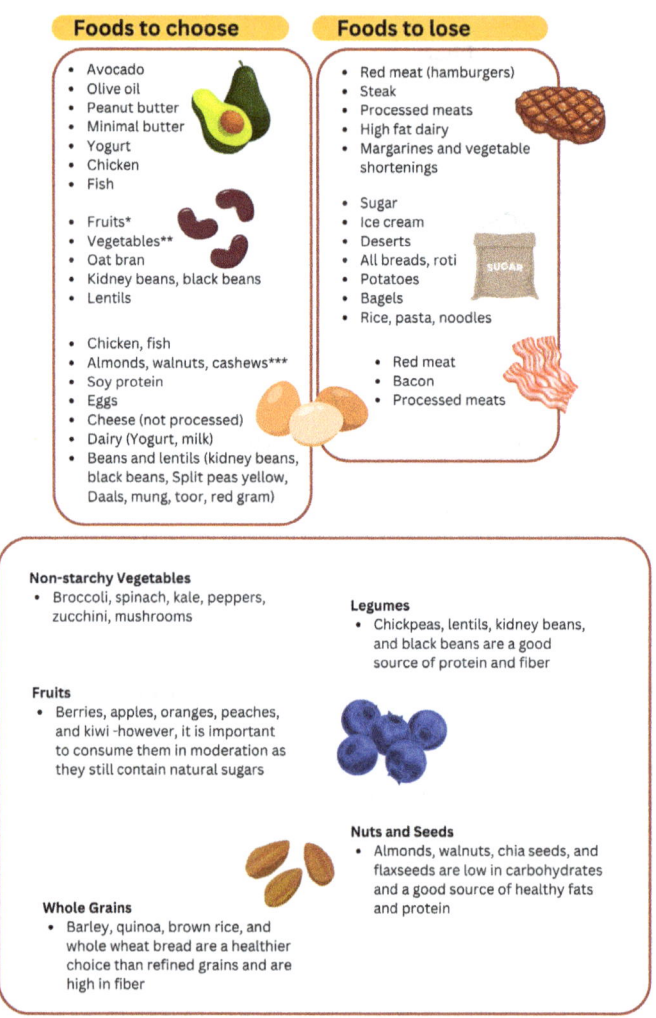

Figure 1: SAHARA© low carbohydrate diet tailored for South Asians and South Asian vegetarians.
*Choose a variety of fruits and variety of colour each day
**Exclude potatoes, and limit corn, eat a variety of vegetables by colour and raw/lightly cooked are preferred
***Non-roasted and non-salted

Low carbohydrate diets are most suited for South Asians as they bring about fat loss and sometimes lead to improvements in lipids, blood sugar, and blood pressure. The challenge for South Asian vegetarians is that vegetarian diets are by design are higher in carbohydrate, so it is even more difficult to initiate and maintain such a diet. In these circumstances increases in non meat-based proteins and good fats are required. In a study we conducted called SAHARA, I designed a low carbohydrate diet tailored for South Asians and South Asian vegetarians (Figure 1). You will see the good non-meat sources of fat and protein required to increase and the low quality carbohydrates to "lose" from the typical diet.

The hardest components of a regular South Asian diet to give up include staples such as basmati rice and roti or naan. These are often staples of the South Asian diet and are tasty and wonderful accompaniments to daals and sabzis. When I discuss with patients, that they must reduce these foods substantially, most feel this is a next to impossible request. A good start is to reduce portion and or size by half, for example if a typical evening meal includes two chapatis, reduce this to 1 chapati to start with in the first week, and eventually reduce this by dropping one day per week to eventually having chapati, naan, or roti once per week on your "off day". Replacement of white polished rice with brown or par boiled rice is also recommended. Other higher protein grains are a reasonable substitute such as quinoa. Given that risk factors can begin early in life, making these changes to the daily dietary intake is a good idea for parents with young children. This is often difficult for young families, especially multigenerational households to implement.

Our research shows that it takes multiple members of a household to want to make similar health changes for them to be successful. For example, if the grandmother of the household thinks it's too extreme to reduce rice and roti, the mother of the household will usually not be successful in making these changes. The pattern I often observe is "prevention" changes are not implemented until a crisis has occurred which includes, "doctors' orders" upon the discovery of gestational diabetes for pregnant women, or a "new diagnosis of pre-diabetes or diabetes" in non-pregnant adults. But even doctors' orders have limited success because often patients don't "feel" the adverse effects of diabetes or high blood pressure for that matter. This is the tension between the emotional brain and the logical brain. Logic would suggest that carbohydrate reduction is required amongst South Asian families, but traditional family dynamics, and usual routines are difficult to break. My advice is **not to wait** until there is a crisis – and adults in the home should be educated on the do's and don'ts, and measure their weight daily – aiming for "their lifetime weight" and then maintaining it +/- 2 pounds for life. However, I recommend rather than making radical dietary changes all at once, a gradual reduction of some undesirable foods, and slow introduction of desirable foods is the optimal approach.

When eating carbohydrates choose **Low glycemic carbohydrates**. David Jenkins and colleagues (1981; 2021) from University of Toronto shift the focus from all carbohydrates are unhealthy to prioritizing low glycemic index (GI) carbs when choosing carbohydrates. The GI, which only measures how quickly a carbohydrate-containing food raises blood sugar levels, the GL takes into account the portion size of the food being eaten. Jenkins' dietary recommendations involve choosing carbohydrates with a low GI, such as fruits, vegetables, and whole grains, while avoiding highly processed foods with added sugars. He also emphasizes the importance of including healthy sources of protein and good fats, such as nuts, seeds, and fish, while limiting intake of saturated and trans fats (Jenkins et al., 2021).

The most striking example of the hazards of any extreme diet came to my attention when I was speaking at a conference on South Asian heart health, and I promoted the utility of a low carbohydrate diet for South Asians. A family doctor approached me at the break and said she had observed one of her patients, South Asian origin, who took this advice so seriously that he developed a B12 deficiency due to such a low carbohydrate consumption that he developed a neurologic condition that affected his balance. While this extreme outcome is rare, it drives home the point that when you choose a diet plan for weight loss you must avoid making radical dietary changes all at once, rather you should make dietary changes in moderation which are likely to be more sustainable and have less adverse effects. However, don't let your mind trick you and remember:

Simple processed carbohydrates with low fiber and/or foods high in added sugar are not healthy, will result in abdominal obesity, possibly diabetes and abnormal lipids, and should be avoided.

Gut Microbiome:
There is emerging research which suggests there has been a missing piece of the puzzle with respect to food intake, digestion, absorption, and circulating by-products in the blood reflecting these processes. The gut microbi-

ome refers to the bacteria that line the small and large intestine. The gut microbiome or flora can be made up of many different types of gut bacteria. These bacteria maybe a higher proportion versus a lower proportion when we compare one individual to the next. There are healthy profiles of gut bacteria and now emerging data suggesting unhealthy profiles of gut bacteria. The proportions of healthy to unhealthy bacteria can then determine if an individual has a severe gastrointestinal disease such as inflammatory bowel disease, or subtle changes in absorption and by-product creation sometimes referred to as the 'gut metabolome'. This missing piece of the puzzle is important when we consider dietary recommendations to prevent cardiovascular risk factors and disease. Because the same food consumed by a different person with a different gut profile may lead to different nutrients being produced and circulating in the body. For example, research from Israel nicely showed that the consumption of a banana by one person can lead to a very different glucose concentration in the bloodstream compared to another person - this between person variability in blood glucose concentration when the same food is consumed may be accounted for in part by variations gut flora (Zeevi et al., 2015). For this reason, we can advise on 'general dietary principles' that may be associated with lower risk of CV risk factors but without knowing the missing piece of the puzzle we cannot generate a "personalized dietary recommendation". The term "personalized nutrition" is gaining traction and may actually become the norm in the future whereby submitting a blood sample, a stool sample, and dietary records may be processed through machine learning or AI algorithms to give personalized dietary recommendations for health to each individual (Cohen et al., 2023; Kviatcovsky et al., 2021; Leshem et al., 2020). This is the future.

In our research involving South Asian infants compared to White European infants in Canada, we observed ethnicity and infant feeding practices influence the gut microbiome at 1 year, and that South Asian infants have a higher abundance of lactic acid bacteria (Stearns et al., 2017). Interestingly Lactobacilli break down mainly carbohydrates that are not absorbed by the host. Other studies have shown that consumption of fermented food and animal flesh foods independently influence the gut microbiome. Comparisons of South Asians from India to Democratic Republic of Congo (DRC) where the diet differs from rice, sorghum, legumes, and buffalo milk in India, to fermented yellow maize porridge, cassava root, fruits and vegetables have been made. Both Bifidobacterium and lactobacillus were enriched in the South Asians. Bacterial diversity was greater in DRC (Tang et al., 2019). The age at which the microbiome becomes mature and persistent is still not well characterized, is it age 1, or does it change all the way up to age 5 years?

Weight Loss:
Some of us come to the realization that we are overweight and must lose 10 to 15 pounds before we can plan to maintain our lifetime weight. There are many **weight loss diets** from which to choose, and no doubt there will be more "must try" diets which emerge in the future. While the principles and targets vary the outcomes are similar. Low carbohydrate diets when compared to low fat diets result in similar weight loss over time, yet low carbohydrate diets are associated with more favourable changes in cardiometabolic risk factors such as reduced triglycerides and some lipoproteins (Foster et al., 2010). Supported by a meta-analyses, a recent comparison of diets tested in randomized trials and published in the New England Journal of Medicine supported this observation (Wadden et al., 2011). Among obese patients in primary care practices, the mean weight loss (±SE) with usual care, brief lifestyle counseling, and enhanced brief lifestyle counseling (including addition of weight loss medications) was 1.7±0.7, 2.9±0.7, and 4.6±0.7 kg, respectively (Wadden et al., 2011). There are now more than 25 randomized trials showing the effectiveness of lowering carbohydrate intake on weight loss (Silverii et al., 2022). The physiologic changes which accompany this weight loss include a reduction in visceral and liver fat, improved lipids, lower blood glucose, and blood pressure. The impact of diet on these parameters is greater, than those which occur through increased physical activity alone, and when combined **low carbohydrate diet** and **increased physical activity** individuals derive the greatest cardiometabolic benefits.

Recently there has been a lot of interest in **intermittent fasting**, which can be adopted in many ways. The 5:2 plan refers to 5 days of normal eating without restriction interspersed with 2 days of fasting (de Cabo & Mattson, 2019). This program is associated with 4-8% body weight loss and many positive changes to metabolic risk markers such as blood cholesterol, glucose and blood pressure. Other intermittent fasting protocols include the **time restricted eating (TRE)** when individuals eat within a time restricted window for example 4-8 hour window, and alternate day fasting. All of these diets lead to weight loss, which peak after 12 weeks of initiation, with the least weight loss observed with the TRE. **Alternate day fasting and 5:2 are also effective at maintain weight and preventing regain**

beyond 12 weeks (Varady et al., 2022). The beneficial effect of intermittent fasting are correlated with changes in gene expression with their feeding schedules in mice (Deota et al., 2023).

Weight loss associated with TRE when compared to caloric restriction (25% reduction from usual caloric intake) irrespective of the timing of eating is similar – pointing to the amount of caloric reduction (Liu et al., 2022), and for some, the type of calories being key drivers of weight loss.

Another program which provides significant resources and has a strong rationale behind it is the "Always Hungry Solution?" created by endocrinologist David Ludwig. There are many resources available to help you kick start your weight loss (see Figure 3), and then your lifelong effort must turn to maintaining your **weight for life** with a low glycemic low carbohydrate diet as your new normal. If you find this impossible to achieve, or are in a high-risk period where you don't have time to wait e.g. your doctor confirms you have type 2 diabetes and other cardiovascular risk factors, you may need to initiate medication treatment, with an oral or an injectable medication for weight loss, or consider bariatric surgery (both described in more detail in Chapter 7).

1. **Health-care providers** e.g. dietitian, doctor, diabetes educator, pharmacist
2. **Health Canada:** https://www.canada.ca/en/services/health/food-nutrition.html
3. **Obesity Canada:** https://obesitycanada.ca/
4. **American Heart Association:** https://www.heart.org/en/
5. **Diabetes Canada:** https://www.diabetes.ca
6. **Centres for Disease Control and Prevention:** https://www.cdc.gov/healthyweight/index.html

Figure 3: Resources to kickstart weight-loss journey

A special note on the importance of regular and sufficient on your health. Shift work with sleep disruption is common amongst healthcare professionals, truck drivers, police or fire officers, and factory workers. **Shift work** causes **chronic disruption of the circadian rhythms** increases the risk of obesity and other metabolic diseases. This makes it even more challenging to maintain a healthy body weight. What can you do to minimize this risk? The first obvious fix is to change your shift work to ensure you have a regular nights sleep. This solution however is not always possible to make– and some of us face this disrupted sleep for years - often when starting out in our careers. I faced this in my medical training, where every 3rd or 4th night we were on-call at the hospital and usually awake all night. I recall drinking coffee throughout the night and also eating comfort foods such as donuts, ordering in pizza, and raiding the vending machines for chocolate bars. Each time I went to see a new patient on the ward after midnight, the nurses had an evening spread of foods to keep us all going – and I relied on that stress relieving sugary fix, mixed with coffee to stay awake. This for certain is not a healthy practice, and studies show disrupted sleep disrupts your neurohormones, and can lead to weight gain which sets off a cascade of other cardiometabolic risk factors.

Another challenging life situation includes **being a parent and raising children** in the North American environment. I know the temptations and satisfaction driven by the children's demand to consume simple sugars, be it at birthday parties, soda pop, and other desserts. Children are typically exposed to these sugars early in life and ask for them repeatedly. Parents who are familiar with the principles of keeping sugar out of diet should try their best to minimize sugar intake in the home. We have also shown that when pregnant South Asian women who consumed sugar sweetened beverages in pregnancy – their children consume also more sugar sweetened beverages (Limbachia et al., 2023). This is an area where we can do better through prevention, though it is not easy to do, especially when both parents are busy working outside the home, and cooking less.

In the UK, where South Asians are the largest non-white ethnic group, they **"are 2-6 times more likely to develop type 2 diabetes and report a higher complication and mortality rate than other population groups"** (Iqbal, 2023). A recent scoping review of South Asians dietary cultural practices in relationship to type 2 diabetes which included detailed review of 19 studies from the UK, indicated that there is a **lack of culturally appropriate advice regarding diet** which is the underlying cause of South Asians' inability to make healthier changes in a sustainable fashion (Iqbal, 2023). There are also strong cultural norms regarding food – "significance of food in creating identity amongst groups of people and therefore, to refuse it, is to lose identity", that if one doesn't follow, can lead to stigmatization by the cultural community (Iqbal, 2023). It also indicated that "adequate education" surrounding the consequences and benefits of diet in T2DM may be effective at mitigating the effects of the deeply ingrained food culture in the South Asian community, and so efforts should focus on **increasing awareness both before and after diagnosis**. It also highlights a high regard given to healthcare professionals by South Asians as they may adopt this advice in defiance of cultural dietary practices. **Healthcare professionals are therefore key actors** in supporting health eating behaviours in the South Asian community (Iqbal, 2023).

One of my colleagues performed an intervention in Ontario, Canada whereby pregnant South Asian women at risk of gestational diabetes were counseled and taught the family doctor who provided them with recipes of healthy meals they could prepare at the end of the study (Kandasamy et al., 2024). Both the family doctor and the pregnant women in the study appreciated the recipes and the beautiful pictures that accompanied them, *but did not act upon them because most of the South Asian women in the study did not cook!* (Kandasamy et al., 2024) They either relied on their mother in laws to drop off food or ordered Tiffin services to deliver food, and in some cases when neither of these were possible, they ate convenience foods given that they were busy caring for other children, or working at the same time (Kandasamy et al., 2024). So again, there is a challenge between *knowing what to eat and what is healthy, and actually being able to do it* and this is where knowledge is the first step, but building in facilitators to healthy active living must be arranged in each family situation on an individual basis – with the mantra *"Make the healthy choice the easy choice."*

A recent study we conducted in Ontario, Canada asked parents of young families of South Asian origin what the barriers and facilitators they faced to healthy active living, and they are listed the following table (Mirza et al., 2022).

Supplementary Table 4 – Member Checking Results
Summary of General Member Checking N = 15

Healthy Eating Barriers		
Not devoting enough time to food preparation	10 agree	5 disagree
Lack of knowledge about what *is* healthy eating	10 agree	5 disagree
Viewing healthy eating as a time-limited challenge, solvable in a few weeks or months	10 agree	5 disagree
Spouse or children's unhealthy eating habits	6 agree	9 disagree
Social pressure to eat traditional, unhealthy foods	6 agree	9 disagree
Healthy Eating Facilitators		
More knowledge about & reminders of what healthy eating is	14 agree	1 disagree
Setting clear goals for eating in a healthier way	14 agree	1 disagree
Better access to fresh vegetables & fruit	14 agree	1 disagree
Clearer arrangements & better tools for healthy food preparation	13 agree	2 disagree
Becoming a vegan or vegetarian	7 agree	8 disagree
Healthy Exercise Barriers		
Not enough time/energy to exercise as other personal priorities are more important	14 agree	1 disagree
Lack of having good childcare (while exercising)	10 agree	5 disagree
Not enough exercise programming that engages my whole family	13 agree	2 disagree
Not enough exercise programming that's interesting, fun and beneficial	7 agree	8 disagree
Healthy Exercise Facilitators		
Experiencing exercise as enjoyable and/or stress releasing	15 agree	0 disagree
Making a committment to walk 'somewhere'	14 agree	1 disagree
Hearing success stories from others who adopt healthy exercise	14 agree	1 disagree
Having a fitbit or other wearable device	13 agree	2 disagree
Being able to exercise with others (including family members)	11 agree	4 disagree

Table 2: Agreement and disagreement among South Asian study participants around common barriers and facilitators to healthy active living (N=15) (Mirza et al., 2022).

In addition, when we analyzed randomized control trials that have assessed the impact of changing diet and physical activity on outcomes such as diabetes, cholesterol, and obesity, and looked at the components of healthy active living that have the greatest impact, we observed that it is **dietary changes** that have the greatest impact on reducing adiposity, and subsequently on cardiovascular risk factors rather than physical activity alone. (Limbachia et al., 2022)

When we place these data in the context of larger studies the data converge on the following take-home messages:
1. Diet has a greater impact on weight and associated metabolic factors more so than physical activity, although when used together physical activity changes augments the impact of dietary changes.
2. Physical activity alone without dietary modification can result in loss of weight but this is relatively limited.
3. When low carbohydrate diet (plus/minus) regular physical activity was evaluated in people who had visceral adipose (fat) tissue on MRI and fatty liver, the first changes in response to these diets occur in the reduction of fat in the liver and visceral fat.

4. Reduction of this fat had a positive effect on cardiometabolic risk factors such as lipids, inflammatory markers, and glucose (Gepner et al., 2018).
5. Physical activity added to the low carbohydrate diet effect on fat reduction, but had lower impact compared to dietary changes alone.

Thus, all the learning to date would show prevention is crucial and it's very difficult for people once they have gained adipose (fat) tissue over 10 to 20 years of time, to first lose it, and then keep it off. The second point, if one has a diagnosis of excess adipose (fat) tissue, glucose, or cholesterol abnormalities there are effective lifestyle ways to alter these risk factors before considering medical treatment. The decision to begin medical treatment to change risk factors should be done together with your physician, but as a clinician practicing for over 25 years, I have observed that patients who have not yet suffered from heart disease, or do not yet have diabetes, would rather try, and change their risk factor profile through lifestyle changes first, before taking a medication(s). These strategies should include consumption of low glycemic carbohydrates, avoiding simple sugars, trying intermittent fasting, and adding in regular physical activity in the form of walking or light aerobic activity, along with light strength training.

We recently showed this by summarizing randomized trials conducted in South Asians. This study aimed to assess the effectiveness of lifestyle interventions in reducing cardiovascular disease risk factors in South Asian populations. The study included 35 studies with ≥90% South Asian participants. The study found that lifestyle interventions, including diet and physical activity, improved blood pressure and blood lipid profiles in adult South Asians at risk of CVD. We concluded that tailored interventions should be used to modify cardiovascular risk factors in this high-risk group. (Limbachia et al., 2022).

Table 3 Comparison 1: diet and physical activity versus usual care (main outcomes)

Outcomes	Anticipated absolute effects* (95% CI)		Relative effect (95% CI)	Participants, n (studies)	Certainty of the evidence (GRADE)
	Risk with usual care	Risk with diet+physical			
SBP (mm Hg)	The mean SBP was 130.63 mm Hg.	MD 2.72 mm Hg lower (from 4.11 lower to 1.33 lower)	–	14 589 (12 RCTs)	⊕⊕⊕◯ Moderate†
SBP (mm Hg), no medications	The mean SBP, no medications, was 127.4 mm Hg.	MD 1.72 mm Hg lower (from 3.71 lower to 0.27 higher)	–	11 715 (5 RCTs)	⊕⊕⊕⊕ High
SBP (mm Hg), medications	The mean SBP, medications, was 133.86 mm Hg.	MD 3.61 mm Hg lower (from 5.63 lower to 1.59 lower)	–	2874 (7 RCTs)	⊕⊕⊕◯ Moderate‡
DBP (mm Hg)	The mean DBP was 85.39 mm Hg.	MD 1.53 mm Hg lower (from 2.57 lower to 0.48 lower)	–	14 527 (11 RCTs)	⊕⊕◯◯ Low§¶
DBP (mm Hg), no medications	The mean DBP, no medications, was 84.93 mm Hg.	MD 0.67 mm Hg lower (from 2.36 lower to 1.01 higher)	–	11 653 (4 RCTs)	⊕⊕⊕◯ Moderate**
DBP (mm Hg), medications	The mean DBP, medications, was 85.85 mm Hg.	MD 2.05 mm Hg lower (from 3.35 lower to 0.75 lower)	–	2874 (7 RCTs)	⊕⊕⊕◯ Moderate¶
Hypertension (yes/no)	34 per 1000	16 per 1000 (6–46)	RR 0.47 (0.17–1.35)	635 (2 RCTs)	⊕⊕⊕◯ Moderate‡‡
Incidence of diabetes (yes/no)	15 per 1000	18 per 1000 (6–60)	RR 1.25 (0.39–4.06)	661 (2 RCTs)	⊕⊕⊕◯ Moderate‡‡

*The **risk in the intervention group** (and its 95% confidence interval) is based on the assumed risk in the comparison group and the **relative effect** of the intervention (and its 95% CI).
*I^2 statistic=54%, p=0.01, implying significant heterogeneity between studies without a lot of overlap in CIs.
†I^2 statistic=58%, p=0.03, implying significant heterogeneity between studies without a lot of overlap in CIs.
‡I^2 statistic=67%, p=0.0008, implying significant heterogeneity between studies without a lot of overlap in CIs.
§Egger's test: p=0.013.
¶I^2 statistic=61%, p=0.02, implying significant heterogeneity between studies without a lot of overlap in CIs.
**I^2 statistic=69%, p=0.02, implying significant heterogeneity between studies without a lot of overlap in CIs.
††Optimal Information Size (OIS) not met.
CI, confidence interval; DBP, diastolic blood pressure; MD, mean difference; RCT, randomised controlled trial; RR, relative risk; SBP, systolic blood pressure.

Figure 5: Table comparing the effects of diet and physical activity on blood pressure and risk of diabetes (Reprinted from Limbachia et al., 2022).

When all else fails, or you are unable to make diet and exercise changes in your life at a crucial time for your health, consider medical therapy to aid in bringing about adipose (fat) tissue – this decision needs to be made together with your doctor.

REFERENCES

Cohen, Y., Valdés-Mas, R., & Elinav, E. (2023). The Role of Artificial Intelligence in Deciphering Diet–Disease Relationships: Case Studies. Annual Review of Nutrition, 43(1), null. https://doi.org/10.1146/annurev-nutr-061121-090535

de Cabo, R., & Mattson, M. P. (2019). Effects of Intermittent Fasting on Health, Aging, and Disease. New England Journal of Medicine, 381(26), 2541–2551. https://doi.org/10.1056/NEJMra1905136

de Koning, L., Merchant, A. T., Pogue, J., & Anand, S. S. (2007). Waist circumference and waist-to-hip ratio as predictors of cardiovascular events: Meta-regression analysis of prospective studies. European Heart Journal, 28(7), 850–856. https://doi.org/10.1093/eurheartj/ehm026

Deota, S., Lin, T., Chaix, A., Williams, A., Le, H., Calligaro, H., Ramasamy, R., Huang, L., & Panda, S. (2023). Diurnal transcriptome landscape of a multi-tissue response to time-restricted feeding in mammals. Cell Metabolism, 35(1), 150-165.e4. https://doi.org/10.1016/j.cmet.2022.12.006

Foster, G. D., Wyatt, H. R., Hill, J. O., Makris, A. P., Rosenbaum, D. L., Brill, C., Stein, R. I., Mohammed, B. S., Miller, B., Rader, D. J., Zemel, B., Wadden, T. A., Tenhave, T., Newcomb, C. W., & Klein, S. (2010). Weight and Metabolic Outcomes After 2 Years on a Low-Carbohydrate Versus Low-Fat Diet. Annals of Internal Medicine, 153(3), 147–157. https://doi.org/10.7326/0003-4819-153-3-201008030-00005

Gepner, Y., Shelef, I., Schwarzfuchs, D., Zelicha, H., Tene, L., Yaskolka Meir, A., Tsaban, G., Cohen, N., Bril, N., Rein, M., Serfaty, D., Kenigsbuch, S., Komy, O., Wolak, A., Chassidim, Y., Golan, R., Avni-Hassid, H., Bilitzky, A., Sarusi, B., … Shai, I. (2018). Effect of Distinct Lifestyle Interventions on Mobilization of Fat Storage Pools. Circulation, 137(11), 1143–1157. https://doi.org/10.1161/CIRCULATIONAHA.117.030501

Grimes, C. A., Riddell, L. J., Campbell, K. J., & Nowson, C. A. (2013). Dietary Salt Intake, Sugar-Sweetened Beverage Consumption, and Obesity Risk. Pediatrics, 131(1), 14–21. https://doi.org/10.1542/peds.2012-1628

Imamura, F., O'Connor, L., Ye, Z., Mursu, J., Hayashino, Y., Bhupathiraju, S. N., & Forouhi, N. G. (2016). Consumption of sugar sweetened beverages, artificially sweetened beverages, and fruit juice and incidence of type 2 diabetes: Systematic review, meta-analysis, and estimation of population attributable fraction. British Journal of Sports Medicine, 50(8), 496–504. https://doi.org/10.1136/bjsports-2016-h3576rep

Iqbal, S. (2023). Cultural factors influencing the eating behaviours of type 2 diabetes in the British South-Asian population: A scoping review of the literature. Journal of Global Health Reports, 7, e2023050. https://doi.org/10.29392/001c.84191

Jenkins, D. J. A., Dehghan, M., Mente, A., Bangdiwala, S. I., Rangarajan, S., Srichaikul, K., Mohan, V., Avezum, A., Díaz, R., Rosengren, A., Lanas, F., Lopez-Jaramillo, P., Li, W., Oguz, A., Khatib, R., Poirier, P., Mohammadifard, N., Pepe, A., Alhabib, K. F., ... Yusuf, S. (2021). Glycemic Index, Glycemic Load, and Cardiovascular Disease and Mortality. New England Journal of Medicine, 384(14), 1312–1322. https://doi.org/10.1056/NEJMoa2007123

Jenkins, D. J., Wolever, T. M., Taylor, R. H., Barker, H., Fielden, H., Baldwin, J. M., Bowling, A. C., Newman, H. C., Jenkins, A. L., & Goff, D. V. (1981). Glycemic index of foods: A physiological basis for carbohydrate exchange. The American Journal of Clinical Nutrition, 34(3), 362–366. https://doi.org/10.1093/ajcn/34.3.362

Kandasamy, S., Amjad, S., de Souza, R., Furqan, N., Patel, T., Vanstone, M., & Anand, S. S. (2024). Getting a "SMART START" to gestational diabetes mellitus education: A mixed-methods pilot evaluation of a knowledge translation tool in primary care. Family Practice, cmad119. https://doi.org/10.1093/fampra/cmad119

Kviatcovsky, D., Zheng, D., & Elinav, E. (2021). Gut microbiome and its potential link to personalized nutrition. Current Opinion in Physiology, 22, 100439. https://doi.org/10.1016/j.cophys.2021.05.002

Leshem, A., Segal, E., & Elinav, E. (2020). The Gut Microbiome and Individual-Specific Responses to Diet. mSystems, 5(5), e00665-20. https://doi.org/10.1128/mSystems.00665-20

Limbachia, J., Ajmeri, M., Keating, B. J., de Souza, R. J., & Anand, S. S. (2022). Effects of lifestyle interventions on cardiovascular risk factors in South Asians: A systematic review and meta-analysis. BMJ Open, 12(12), e059666. https://doi.org/10.1136/bmjopen-2021-059666

Limbachia, J., Desai, D., Abdalla, N., de Souza, R. J., Teo, K., Morrison, K. M., Punthakee, Z., Gupta, M., Lear, S. A., Anand, S. S., & for the START, F., and RICH LEGACY Canada Investigators. (2023). The association of maternal sugary beverage consumption during pregnancy and the early years with childhood sugary beverage consumption. Canadian Journal of Public Health, 114(2), 231–240. https://doi.org/10.17269/s41997-022-00681-1

Liu, D., Huang, Y., Huang, C., Yang, S., Wei, X., Zhang, P., Guo, D., Lin, J., Xu, B., Li, C., He, H., He, J., Liu, S., Shi, L., Xue, Y., & Zhang, H. (2022). Calorie Restriction with or without Time-Restricted Eating in Weight Loss. New England Journal of Medicine, 386(16), 1495–1504. https://doi.org/10.1056/NEJMoa2114833

Malik, V. S., Popkin, B. M., Bray, G. A., Després, J.-P., & Hu, F. B. (2010). Sugar-Sweetened Beverages, Obesity, Type 2 Diabetes Mellitus, and Cardiovascular Disease Risk. Circulation, 121(11), 1356–1364. https://doi.org/10.1161/CIRCULATIONAHA.109.876185

Merchant, A., Anand, S. S., Vuksan, V., Jacobs, R., Davis, B., Teo, K., & Yusuf, S. (2005). Protein Intake Is Inversely Associated with Abdominal Obesity in a Multi-Ethnic Population. The Journal of Nutrition, 135(5), 1196–1201. https://doi.org/10.1093/jn/135.5.1196

Merchant, A., Yusuf, S., & Sharma, A. M. (2006). A cardiologist's guide to waist management. Heart, 92(7), 865–866. https://doi.org/10.1136/hrt.2005.080945

Mirza, S., Kandasamy, S., Souza, R. J. de, Wahi, G., Desai, D., Anand, S. S., & Ritvo, P. (2022). Barriers and facilitators to healthy active living in South Asian families in Canada: A thematic analysis. BMJ Open, 12(11), e060385. https://doi.org/10.1136/bmjopen-2021-060385

Pan, L., Li, R., Park, S., Galuska, D. A., Sherry, B., & Freedman, D. S. (2014). A Longitudinal Analysis of Sugar-Sweetened Beverage Intake in Infancy and Obesity at 6 Years. Pediatrics, 134(Supplement_1), S29–S35. https://doi.org/10.1542/peds.2014-0646F

Silverii, G. A., Cosentino, C., Santagiuliana, F., Rotella, F., Benvenuti, F., Mannucci, E., & Cresci, B. (2022). Effectiveness of low-carbohydrate diets for long-term weight loss in obese individuals: A meta-analysis of randomized controlled trials. Diabetes, Obesity and Metabolism, 24(8), 1458–1468. https://doi.org/10.1111/dom.14709

Stearns, J. C., Zulyniak, M. A., de Souza, R. J., Campbell, N. C., Fontes, M., Shaikh, M., Sears, M. R., Becker, A. B., Mandhane, P. J., Subbarao, P., Turvey, S. E., Gupta, M., Beyene, J., Surette, M. G., Anand, S. S., & for the NutriGen Alliance. (2017). Ethnic and diet-related differences in the healthy infant microbiome. Genome Medicine, 9(1), 32. https://doi.org/10.1186/s13073-017-0421-5

Tang, M., Frank, D. N., Tshefu, A., Lokangaka, A., Goudar, S. S., Dhaded, S. M., Somannavar, M. S., Hendricks, A. E., Ir, D., Robertson, C. E., Kemp, J. F., Lander, R. L., Westcott, J. E., Hambidge, K. M., & Krebs, N. F. (2019). Different Gut Microbial Profiles in Sub-Saharan African and South Asian Women of Childbearing Age Are Primarily Associated With Dietary Intakes. Frontiers in Microbiology, 10. https://www.frontiersin.org/articles/10.3389/fmicb.2019.01848

Varady, K. A., Cienfuegos, S., Ezpeleta, M., & Gabel, K. (2022). Clinical application of intermittent fasting for weight loss: Progress and future directions. Nature Reviews Endocrinology, 18(5), Article 5. https://doi.org/10.1038/s41574-022-00638-x

Wadden, T. A., Volger, S., Sarwer, D. B., Vetter, M. L., Tsai, A. G., Berkowitz, R. I., Kumanyika, S., Schmitz, K. H., Diewald, L. K., Barg, R., Chittams, J., & Moore, R. H. (2011). A Two-Year Randomized Trial of Obesity Treatment in Primary Care Practice. New England Journal of Medicine, 365(21), 1969–1979. https://doi.org/10.1056/NEJMoa1109220

Wang, M., Yu, M., Fang, L., & Hu, R.-Y. (2015). Association between sugar-sweetened beverages and type 2 diabetes: A meta-analysis. Journal of Diabetes Investigation, 6(3), 360–366. https://doi.org/10.1111/jdi.12309

Zeevi, D., Korem, T., Zmora, N., Israeli, D., Rothschild, D., Weinberger, A., Ben-Yacov, O., Lador, D., Avnit-Sagi, T., Lotan-Pompan, M., Suez, J., Mahdi, J. A., Matot, E., Malka, G., Kosower, N., Rein, M., Zilberman-Schapira, G., Dohnalová, L., Pevsner-Fischer, M., ... Segal, E. (2015). Personalized Nutrition by Prediction of Glycemic Responses. Cell, 163(5), 1079–1094. https://doi.org/10.1016/j.cell.2015.11.001

Chapter 5
What about physical activity?

Just like patients who receive a prescription to start taking cholesterol medication, I often write in clinic a healthy active living prescription for healthy diet and regular exercise, so patients take them as seriously as their prescription medications.

What do we mean by physical activity?

Physical activity is activity that increases one's heart rate and breathing rate and can lead to perspiration. Activities that we do that bring this on be it housecleaning to jogging to playing soccer are referred to as physical activity. **The most common form of activity is walking, brisk walking, walking with a heavy load, walking uphill, or walking up stairs and all count as physical activity.** In high income countries where weight gain is a common consequence of an urban lifestyle and sedentary jobs, adults who are health conscious try to join a gym, take on a running club, or run a marathon. In other countries such as India especially in rural areas, or for those with manual labour jobs which are physically taxing - "leisure-time" exercise is not something to think about because the days' work is so physically onerous.

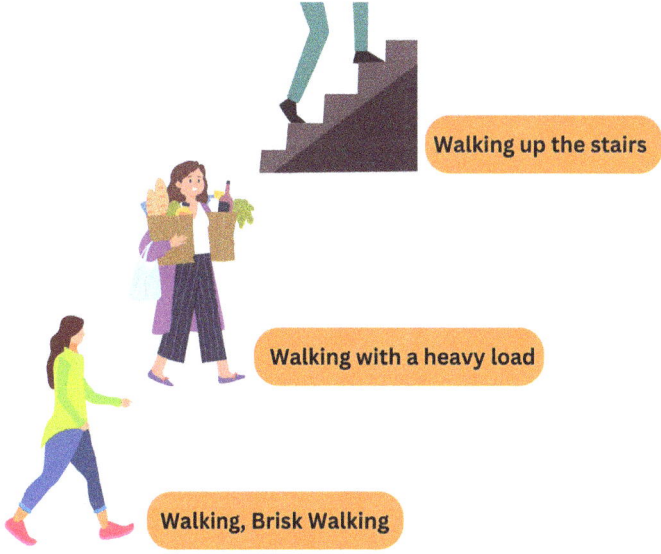

Regular physical activity has been a part of a healthy mode of living for centuries as indicated in the Ayurvedic Texts. The World Health Organization (WHO) reports that over a quarter of the global adult population does not engage in sufficient physical activity in 2022 (WHO, 2024). Physical activity levels are drastically different comparing rural India to urban India and urban North America. Specifically, individuals in rural areas tend to engage in higher levels of physical activity compared to those in urban areas of India. This is primarily due to the nature of occupations in rural regions, which often involve more manual labor and physical tasks. In Canada the SAHARA randomized trial along with other evaluations have generally shown South Asians in North American perform lower levels of physical activity compared to their counterparts in rural India (Anand et al., 2016; Fernando et al., 2015; Lear et al., 2017).

In parallel the minutes we used to expend being active have been replaced by minutes spent sitting usually in front of computer screens. The average office worker or person "working from home" spends 6-8 hours per day in front of a computer usually sitting. Furthermore, trying to make up for the time spent sitting by doing an aggressive "work-out" doesn't compensate - the recommendation is to stand at your desk, and to interrupt sitting screen time with walks around your building or local neighbourhood.

A typical North American day in cities not designed for walking is reflective of the sedentary life that many of us lead – driving to work, sitting in front of a computer screen 8-hours of work, and then driving home, followed by eating, reclining, or lying on the couch, and again watching our screens on a laptop or flat-screen television in our leisure time. Recognizing the time spent sitting and time spent in front of a screen in totality is very informative - many health studies have measured both sedentary and time spent being active, exercising. There are many wide spread benefits of regular physical activity on cardio-metabolic processes (Ashcroft et al., 2024).

Here is what we know about physical activity and sedentary times effect on health. 10,000 steps per day is a commonly recommended physical activity goal that can have several health benefits.

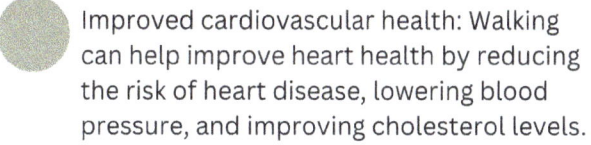

Some of the potential health benefits of walking 10,000 steps per day include:

- Improved cardiovascular health: Walking can help improve heart health by reducing the risk of heart disease, lowering blood pressure, and improving cholesterol levels.

- Weight management: Walking can help with weight loss or maintenance by burning calories and increasing metabolism.

- Improved mental health: Physical activity, including walking, can help improve mood and reduce symptoms of depression and anxiety.

Often, we think of and hear in the media that our fat stores are directly related to a "calories in calories out" calculation, but in the previous chapter I reviewed how the type of calories also matter when we think about health. Physical activity and sedentary behaviours are the two factors which also impact our propensity to increased body fat. For South Asians that means the Canadian Tire which appears at key times in our lives: 1) men in their early 20s when they become less active no longer doing school-based sports or university intramurals, 2) women this becomes noticeable after each successive pregnancy with weight retention typically in the order of five to 10 pounds per pregnancy, and 3) after age 50 for adults who have "gained a pound a year" – this insidious weight gain especially among women after the menopause. How then should we think about physical activity and minimizing sedentary behaviors to minimize the chance of our developing a Canadian Tire?

Just like patients who receive a prescription to start taking cholesterol medication, I often write in clinic a healthy active living prescription for healthy diet, regular exercise, and resistance training, so patients take them as seriously as their other medications.

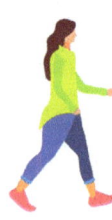

30mins of brisk walking per day

Use a step counter or phone app
(10, 000 steps/day)

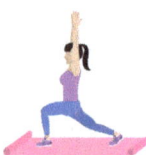

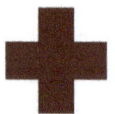

| Pilates | Light arm weight | Trainer at the gym (3 times/week) |

30 minutes of brisk walking per day (as a minimum); or regular sports such as tennis, squash, cross country skiing, swimming

Use a step counter or phone app to track **10,000 steps per day**

Stand up and walk around the office or the home once each hour

Strength training with light weight or power yoga to maintain muscle mass

Ideally a lifelong love of healthy active living can be inculcated in all children from a young age - this outdoor activity, organized sports, or daily yoga and fitness practice, would ideally take hold and stay with the individual long term. In South Asian culture and sub-cultures there are the added challenges of gender-based stigma around playing sports and developing visible muscles. Proactive parents should recognize that optimizing the health of their families begins with a strong recognition and endorsement of the importance of minimizing ultra processed foods and maximizing activities for families to preserve good health of parents and their children.

> Parents should also recognize that physical activity has other positive spin-offs - including improved school performance, lower bullying, and improved mental health and wellness.

In high income countries like Canada, we have winter and summer sports, and we have many opportunities in school for children to play them. However, in university/college and afterwards regular physical activity must become a deliberate practice, or else it won't find a place into our busy lives, especially with marriage and children further competing for adult's time.

The tough part of making regular physical activity a deliberate practice is because in general our workplaces do not make regular exercise easy for us – although this is context dependent. People who live in "walkable cities or neighbourhoods" can walk for errands, walk to work, and/or walk to school. People who choose or are forced to live a long distance from work, errands, and school however have to drive or take transportation everywhere. So much of why we choose a place to live has to do with the house, its price, its space, but often less to do with our health and happiness. Perhaps with the societal reckoning on-going regarding the climate crisis, choosing where to live will land more of us right in the heart of a walkable, beautiful neighbourhood, and car ownership will decline.

Personal trainers, Health Coaches; Social Networks
Should you join a gym, should you join Weight Watchers, should you join other groups that help you to bring about lifestyle changes? It is possible, there is some evidence that social support networks in exercise and in dietary changes are effective, and thus if you have the financial means these

can be effective and can include joining an exercise or weight loss group, or even joining a personal trainer. The Diabetes Prevention Project was a highly successful lifestyle intervention of; 1) individual case managers or "lifestyle coaches;" 2) frequent contact with participants; and 3) a structured, state-of-the-art, 16-session core-curriculum that taught behavioral self-management strategies for weight loss and physical activity; and 4) supervised physical activity sessions (DPP Research Group, 2002). In this randomize clinical trial the lifestyle intervention decreased the incidence of type 2 diabetes by 58% compared to usual care more so that the 31% reduction observed in the metformin-treated group!

Furthermore, resistance training is associated with lower mortality by 21% (Saeidifard et al., 2019). This type of routine may result in weight and fat loss, decrease central obesity, and lead to improvements in cardio metabolic factors (Limbachia et al., 2022).

Sleep, Naps and Rest:
The relationship between sleep and cardiometabolic health is complicated. Non-experimental research studies have shown, too little sleep, and too much sleep are both associated with increased mortality – mostly attributed to cardiovascular causes. The optimal duration of continuous sleep in a 24-hour period appears to be 8 hours – durations < 6 and > 9 are associated with adverse health consequences like diabetes. **Taking naps can be good for your health, especially if you are not getting enough sleep at night. Napping can help you feel more alert and refreshed, and may have several health benefits, including improved thinking ability, immunity boost and lower stress.** Short naps of 20-30 minutes are generally considered ideal, as it can provide a quick energy boost without disrupting nighttime sleep. Shift work – meaning working days and being awake during an individual's usual sleeping hours also has adverse consequences for health. The metabolic pathways which are disrupted affect appetite, signals to the brain, and have been shown to increase blood pressure, cholesterol, body weight, and blood glucose. Shift work has been found to have a negative effect on cholesterol levels. Several studies have shown that working irregular or night shifts is associated with an increased risk of dyslipidemia, which is a condition characterized by abnormal levels of cholesterol and/or triglycerides in the blood. One study published in the journal "Atherosclerosis" in 2016 found that shift workers had higher levels of LDL ("bad") cholesterol and lower levels of HDL ("good") cholesterol compared to non-shift workers. Another study published in "PLOS ONE"

in 2015 found that shift work was associated with an increased risk of metabolic syndrome, a cluster of conditions that includes dyslipidemia as a key component (Guo et al., 2015). Naps (think siestas in Spain, afternoon naps in Greece) in some cultures are considered a normal part of the daily routine. Short duration naps e.g., 20 minutes that are sometimes labelled "power naps" can be beneficial whereas naps beyond that duration can make it difficult for an individual to return to normal pace due to a "hangover" effect and may disrupt night-time sleep.

What I recommend as the Optimal Activity Prescription for Health: Randomized trials or interventions where physical activity was independently evaluated for its impact on body weight, body adiposity, and other risk factors have collectively shown that regular physical activity is associated with improved cardio-metabolic health (Armstrong et al., 2022; Battista et al., 2021). RCTs to reduce sedentary time have shown that interventions introduced in early childhood result in significant decreases in behavior compared to interventions given to adults, suggesting that instilling healthy habits early in life is important (Downing et al., 2018; Shrestha et al., 2019; van Grieken et al., 2012). A systematic review of South Asian specific trials that we conducted showed that regular physical activity was associated with improvements in CVD risk factors, including blood pressure and cholesterol levels– and thus findings are generally consistent with the larger studies conducted in allcomers (Limbachia et al., 2022).

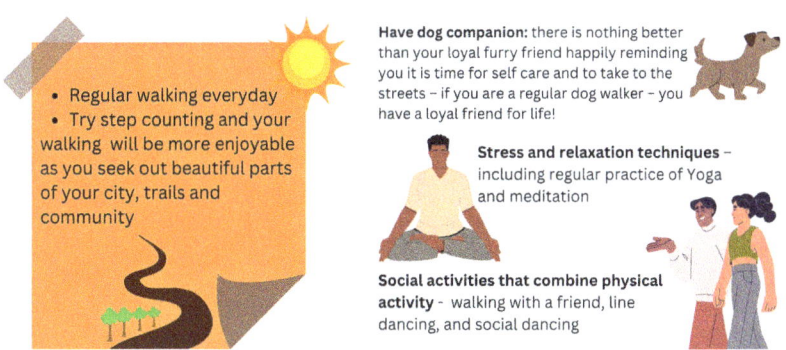

The Diabetes Prevention Project nicely showed addition of a personal trainer to once daily routine as a way to re-enforce and motivate an individual to keep exercising is effective, as did an RCT from Israel showing both low carbohydrate diet and regular physical activity regularly contribute to weight and fat loss, with the change to a low carb diet having the greater impact than the physical activity, but both contributed independently to weight and fat loss (DPP Research Group, 2002; Gepner et al., 2018).

Strength training:
Finally, a note on strength training. Increased muscle mass improves strength, prevents injury, and can improve weight maintenance and certain cardiometabolic processes such as improved glucose control. Muscle mass begins to decline after the age of 50 years so the peak years to build strength are before this. The adage "use it or lose it" applies here too. Modest strength training including push-ups, power yoga, light weights are easy to do with minimal expense. Of course, more elaborate programs are beneficial too albeit sometimes more costly. The greatest barrier to strength training programs is motivation of individuals to maintain them overtime. Social engagement with friends or coworkers around fitness is a good way to maintain exercise programs and keep it enjoyable.

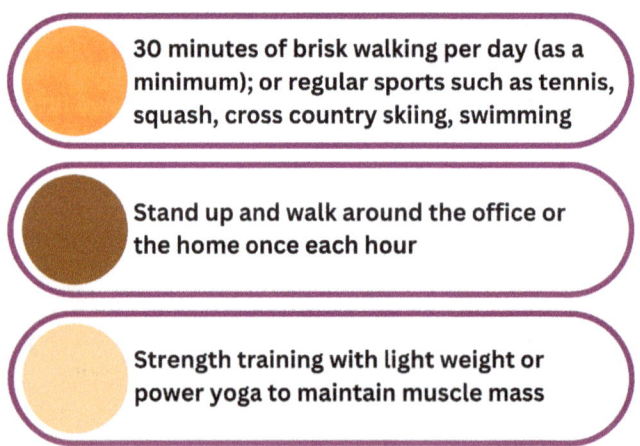

REFERENCES

Anand, S. S., Samaan, Z., Middleton, C., Irvine, J., Desai, D., Schulze, K. M., Sothiratnam, S., Hussain, F., Shah, B. R., Pare, G., Beyene, J., Lear, S. A., & South Asian Heart Risk Assessment Investigators. (2016). A Digital Health Intervention to Lower Cardiovascular Risk: A Randomized Clinical Trial. JAMA Cardiology, 1(5), 601–606. https://doi.org/10.1001/jamacardio.2016.1035

Armstrong, A., Jungbluth Rodriguez, K., Sabag, A., Mavros, Y., Parker, H. M., Keating, S. E., & Johnson, N. A. (2022). Effect of aerobic exercise on waist circumference in adults with overweight or obesity: A systematic review and meta-analysis. Obesity Reviews: An Official Journal of the International Association for the Study of Obesity, 23(8), e13446. https://doi.org/10.1111/obr.13446

Ashcroft, S. P., Stocks, B., Egan, B., & Zierath, J. R. (2024). Exercise induces tissue-specific adaptations to enhance cardiometabolic health. Cell Metabolism. https://doi.org/10.1016/j.cmet.2023.12.008

Battista, F., Ermolao, A., van Baak, M. A., Beaulieu, K., Blundell, J. E., Busetto, L., Carraça, E. V., Encantado, J., Dicker, D., Farpour-Lambert, N., Pramono, A., Bellicha, A., & Oppert, J.-M. (2021). Effect of exercise on cardiometabolic health of adults with overweight or obesity: Focus on blood pressure, insulin resistance, and intrahepatic fat-A systematic review and meta-analysis. Obesity Reviews: An Official Journal of the International Association for the Study of Obesity, 22 Suppl 4(Suppl 4), e13269. https://doi.org/10.1111/obr.13269

Downing, K. L., Hnatiuk, J. A., Hinkley, T., Salmon, J., & Hesketh, K. D. (2018). Interventions to reduce sedentary behaviour in 0-5-year-olds: A systematic review and meta-analysis of randomised controlled trials. British Journal of Sports Medicine, 52(5), 314–321. https://doi.org/10.1136/bjsports-2016-096634

DPP Research Group. (2002). The Diabetes Prevention Program (DPP): Description of lifestyle intervention. Diabetes Care, 25(12), 2165–2171. https://doi.org/10.2337/diacare.25.12.2165

Fernando, E., Razak, F., Lear, S. A., & Anand, S. S. (2015). Cardiovascular Disease in South Asian Migrants. Canadian Journal of Cardiology, 31(9), 1139–1150. https://doi.org/10.1016/j.cjca.2015.06.008

Gepner, Y., Shelef, I., Schwarzfuchs, D., Zelicha, H., Tene, L., Yaskolka Meir, A., Tsaban, G., Cohen, N., Bril, N., Rein, M., Serfaty, D., Kenigsbuch, S., Komy, O., Wolak, A., Chassidim, Y., Golan, R., Avni-Hassid, H., Bilitzky, A., Sarusi, B., ... Shai, I. (2018). Effect of Distinct Lifestyle Interventions on Mobilization of Fat Storage Pools. Circulation, 137(11), 1143–1157. https://doi.org/10.1161/CIRCULATIONAHA.117.030501

Guo, Y., Rong, Y., Huang, X., Lai, H., Luo, X., Zhang, Z., Liu, Y., He, M., Wu, T., & Chen, W. (2015). Shift Work and the Relationship with Metabolic Syndrome in Chinese Aged Workers. PLOS ONE, 10(3), e0120632. https://doi.org/10.1371/journal.pone.0120632

Lear, S. A., Hu, W., Rangarajan, S., Gasevic, D., Leong, D., Iqbal, R., Casanova, A., Swaminathan, S., Anjana, R. M., Kumar, R., Rosengren, A., Wei, L., Yang, W., Chuangshi, W., Huaxing, L., Nair, S., Diaz, R., Swidon, H., Gupta, R., ... Yusuf, S. (2017). The effect of physical activity on mortality and cardiovascular disease in 130 000 people from 17 high-income, middle-income, and low-income countries: The PURE study. Lancet (London, England), 390(10113), 2643–2654. https://doi.org/10.1016/S0140-6736(17)31634-3

Limbachia, J., Ajmeri, M., Keating, B. J., de Souza, R. J., & Anand, S. S. (2022). Effects of lifestyle interventions on cardiovascular risk factors in South Asians: A systematic review and meta-analysis. BMJ Open, 12(12), e059666. https://doi.org/10.1136/bmjopen-2021-059666

Saeidifard, F., Medina-Inojosa, J. R., West, C. P., Olson, T. P., Somers, V. K., Bonikowske, A. R., Prokop, L. J., Vinciguerra, M., & Lopez-Jimenez, F. (2019). The association of resistance training with mortality: A systematic review and meta-analysis. European Journal of Preventive Cardiology, 26(15), 1647–1665. https://doi.org/10.1177/2047487319850718

Shrestha, N., Grgic, J., Wiesner, G., Parker, A., Podnar, H., Bennie, J. A., Biddle, S. J. H., & Pedisic, Z. (2019). Effectiveness of interventions for reducing non-occupational sedentary behaviour in adults and older adults: A systematic review and meta-analysis. British Journal of Sports Medicine, 53(19), 1206–1213. https://doi.org/10.1136/bjsports-2017-098270

van Grieken, A., Ezendam, N. P. M., Paulis, W. D., van der Wouden, J. C., & Raat, H. (2012). Primary prevention of overweight in children and adolescents: A meta-analysis of the effectiveness of interventions aiming to decrease sedentary behaviour. The International Journal of Behavioral Nutrition and Physical Activity, 9, 61. https://doi.org/10.1186/1479-5868-9-61

WHO. (2024, June 26). Physical activity. World Health Organization. https://www.who.int/news-room/fact-sheets/detail/physical-activity

Chapter 6
Surely stress must play a role?

Each time I see a patient and tell them about their risk factors for heart disease or give a presentation to a South Asian audience someone in the room will ask if stress has something to do with the development of abdominal obesity, diabetes, or unexpected heart disease. In my early days as a practitioner and researcher I was quick to say, "most likely no". However, with the passage of time, the experience I have gained seeing many patients, hearing hundreds of personal stories, and carefully following the medical literature – I do believe that stress plays a role in our overall physical health.

First off, I have personally experienced an unexpected cardiac issue for which there really was no cogent explanation other than the extreme stress I had experienced. I had kept the stress bottled up inside, it was the first thing I thought of when I awoke in the morning and last thing I thought about before going to sleep – this on top of my busy medical practice, research demands, and being married with 3 children under the age of 15 years. After about 4 months of this stress "something gave" and I required medical tests and scans to try and get to the bottom of the issue. The advice from my cardiac specialists was to "slow down, and live a more balanced life" and "don't take on so much work with so many deadlines" and "take fewer 'weekend' trips to Europe for work".

Second, while shorter term acute stress like the type I experienced is associated with illness, chronic ongoing stress such as suffering through a difficult marriage, having a challenging time parenting, or leaving all of one's security in one's home country to move thousands of miles to a new country, is associated with illness as well. With all of these stressors sometimes people use food and alcohol as medicine to help diminish the stress. If this response to stress occurs over a long period of time, one can gain 10 to 20 pounds of weight without realizing– until a friend says something, or until your clothes don't fit. Many of my patients have described this to me, they came to Canada in their mid-twenties with a goal of reaching economic success, having enough wealth to own their own home, having a good job, a car, and being able to send their children to good schools. This sometimes expanded to include helping their families back home, and facilitating the immigration of their brothers, sisters, and in-laws. As time in their new country increased, so did their weight. For men this was a gradual increase in girth and on average 1 pound per year. Among women it was usually, post-partum weight retention, of at least 5 pounds after each child was born.

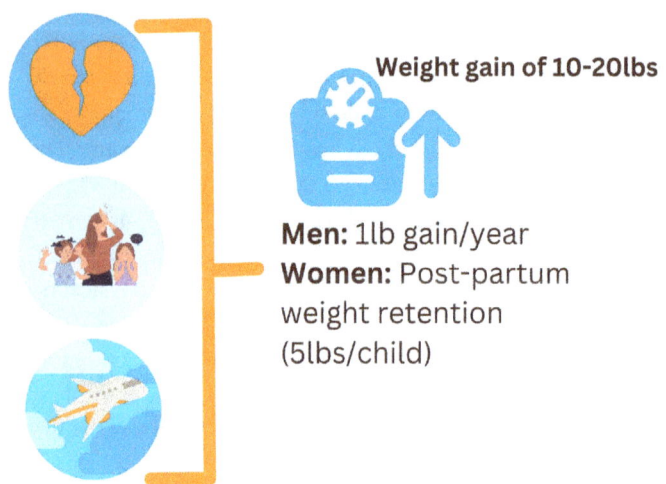

Weight gain of 10-20lbs

Men: 1lb gain/year
Women: Post-partum weight retention (5lbs/child)

Story of migration stress

No discussion of heart disease risk would be complete without our review of the role of how stress is associated with ill health. Often when I would give presentations to South Asian audiences on premature heart disease afflicting South Asians migrants, at question period audience members would convey their belief that "the stress of migration" to another country played a large part of their suffering unexpected cardiac disease. First, there is no doubt that disrupting one's lifestyles is stressful and changes in lifestyles patterns which can have adverse consequences – that is the seed in the soil analogy. However mental stress which occurs with migration can also occur within India or Pakistan when a rural dwelling person migrates to an urban region – because as social networks are disrupted and reformed, and so too are lifestyle factors.

What do we know about stress and heart disease?

How can mental stress be connected to heart disease? Gabor Mate a psychiatrist has written an excellent book called "When the Body says No":

The Costs of Hidden Stress in which he described the body manifests with physical breakdown of systems including cancer, cardiovascular disease, and neurologic manifestations when stress is not processed and managed well (Maté, 2003).

Figure 1 shows a multitude of pathways – and in addition the type of stress can have differential effects on health. Patients often speak of good stress (e.g. being busy in careers they enjoy) and bad stress (e,g. financial worries, interpersonal conflicts etc.). In our research studies we ask about financial, personal stress, strife within families, and how "in control" of one's affairs at work or at home, is the individual. High stress can be correlated with adverse health behaviors such as unhealthy eating, reduced activity, and smoking – and have other unknown relationships to illness. Emotional stress can increase the risk of a heart attack. Emotional stress can trigger the release of stress hormones, such as cortisol and adrenaline, which can cause changes in the body that increase the risk of heart attack. These changes include increased heart rate and blood pressure, which can put additional strain on the heart (Anand et al., 2008; Li et al., 2014; Vahedian-Azimi & Moayed, 2019).

Stress eating is also a well characterized phenomenon which is correlated with various life stressors in particular "work stress", who hasn't been in the situation of coming home after ones work day, with the requirement of picking up the children from activities or school, rushing home, to cook a fresh meal for the family, thereby beginning "work at home", for the second half of the day. Stress eating can occur while cooking and tasting, eating up leftovers, or at the end of the day finding some comfort in eating a sweet treat like ice cream. When the brain experiences stress, it signals the release of hormones, some of which influence appetite and weight. For example, cortisol known as the "stress hormone" leads to increased food intake, whereas insulin the growth hormone signals the body to store energy as fat (Czech et al., 2013; Herhaus et al., 2020). Studies from mice suggest that experiencing stress can lead to increased activity of reward areas of the brain while reducing the effectiveness of control areas, leading to an increase desire to eat certain foods (Ip et al., 2023).

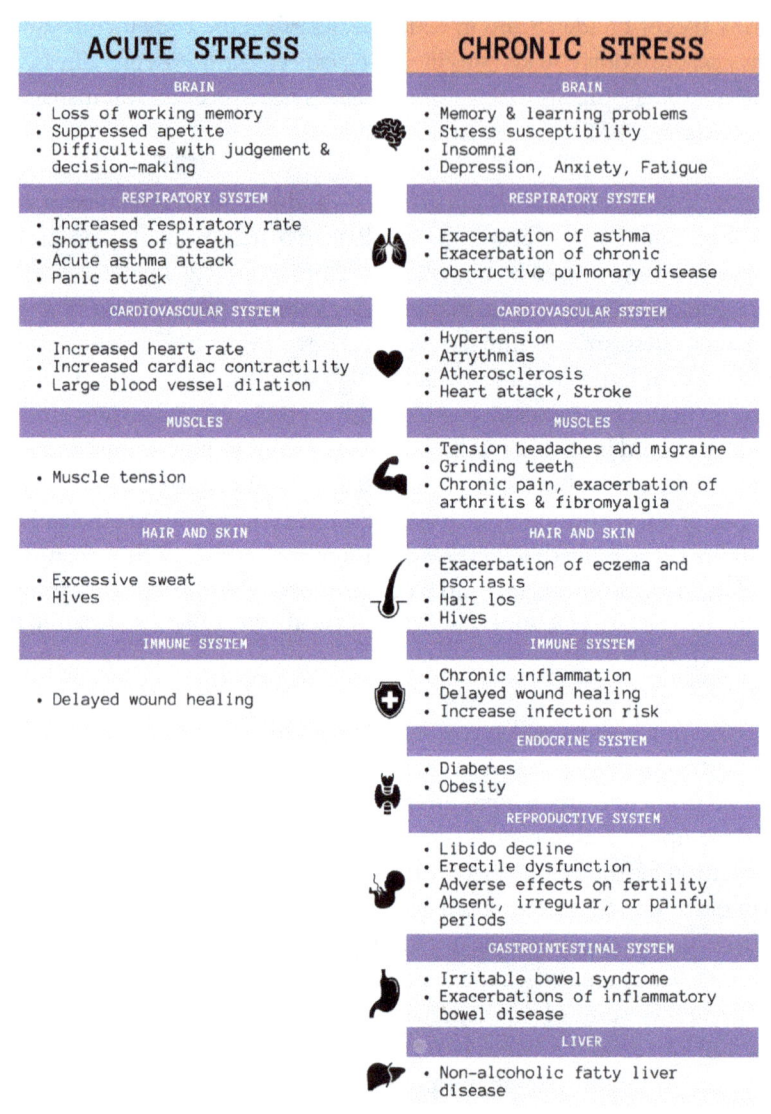

Figure 1: Pathways in which acute and chronic stress affect health (Adapted with permission from Connelly, 2021).

There are many potential stressors in our lives not just work stress, there is family relationship stress, and even community factors involved in stress such as experiencing racism (Bulatao et al., 2004). Furthermore, studies of the general population show our stress responses can cause some of us to undereat (usually related to acute stress), and some of us to overeat (usually in response to a chronic stress), and a minority of people don't change their eating habits in response to stress at all (lucky them!). Comfort foods are usually convenient, ultraprocessed, ready-to-eat foods like chocolate bars, potato chips, or ice-cream, which means they take less effort to prepare, result in a dopamine rush and a feeling of comfort. While it may be fine to indulge in these types of foods occasionally to deal with stress, if they are repeatedly eaten over a long period of time, they are likely to lead to increased weight gain (Torres & Nowson, 2007).

In our interviews of South Asian parents with young children (Mirza et al., 2022), we learned about the main **barriers and facilitators to healthy eating and physical activity**:

BARRIERS TO AND FACILITATORS OF
HEALTHY LIFESTYLES
(MIRZA ET AL., 2022)

BARRIERS TO HEALTHY EATING
- Lack of time for engaging in healthy food preparation
- Lack of knowledge about healthy eating
- Viewing healthy eating as a time-limited diet
- Spouses/children's unhealthy eating habits
- Personal pressures to eat unhealthy foods

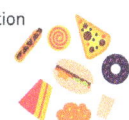

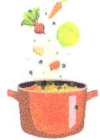

FACILITATORS OF HEALTHY EATING
- Setting clear goals
- Better access to fresh vegetables and fruits
- Clear arrangements for food preparation
- Engaging in vegetarian/vegan ways of eating

BARRIERS TO PHYSICAL ACTIVITY
- Lack of time and energy to engage in exercise, competing priorities
- Lack of childcare
- Limited access to relevant programs

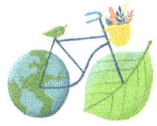

FACILITATORS OF PHYSICAL ACTIVITY
- Viewing exercise as enjoyable and stress releasing
- Use of tracking devices
- Family support

This brings us to the third component, what does the evidence from the medical literature show?

1. There is a substantial evidence base supporting the causal relationship between psychological stress and cardiovascular disease. For instance, chronic stress exposure results in maladaptive immune, endocrine, and metabolic responses.
2. Acute stress-induced inflammation may precipitate atherosclerotic plaque destabilization.

The INTERHEART study was a large case-control study evaluating over 11,000 patients with a first heart attack and over 13,000 age- and sex-matched controls from 52 countries world-wide, showed that participants who had suffered from a heart attack were more than twice as likely to report permanent stress at the workplace (odds ratio 2.12 [99%CI, 1.68–2.93]) compared with people who did not have a history of a heart attack (Lagraauw et al., 2015; Rosengren et al., 2004; Yusuf et al., 2004). Also, more patients with an acute heart attack reported being exposed to two or more acute stressful life events (e.g. loss of a loved one, divorce, loss of job or business failure) in the previous year (odds ratio 1.48 [99%CI, 1.33–1.64]) (Lagraauw et al., 2015; Rosengren et al., 2004).

Furthermore from the INTERHEART study, the lower a person feels in control in their workplace or at home, the higher the risk of heart attack (Rosengren et al., 2004). This points to the chronic nature of stress, and occurs irrespective of social position (Marmot & Brunner, 2005).

Ways to relieve mental stress are described below:
We must accept that stress in life occurs, we also have to accept that the ways in which people respond to stressors is different, and that our responses to stress may affect our eating behaviours, activity patterns, blood pressure, and our risk of heart attack, not to mention other chronic diseases such as diabetes and possibly cancer. Thus, when thinking of stress reducing strategies – these must be tailored to our personality types – meaning a one size fits all approach will not work. We will turn to Ayurveda to understand how stress was described in ancient texts and advice given according to Dosha's in the Chapter 8, but first we will review what the western medicine suggests.

How to manage stress (Strategies with Evidence):

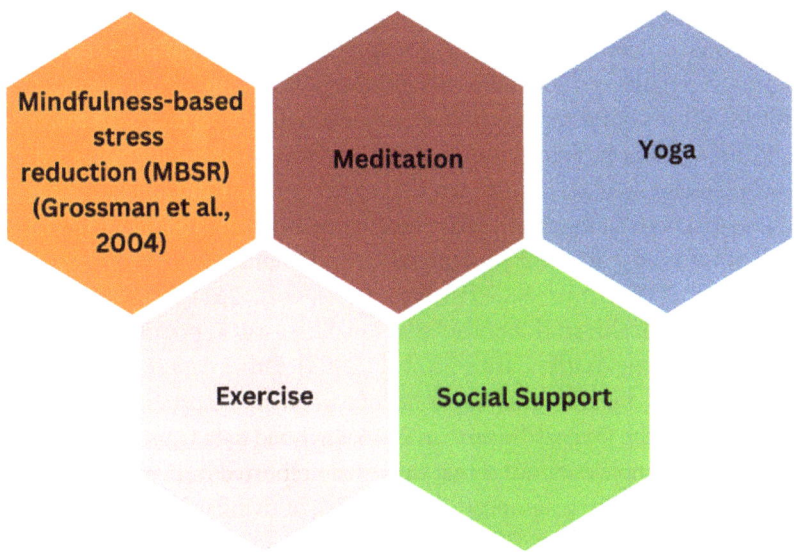

Other Lifestyle Factors:
Most of the material presented in this book has been well tested and characterized from intervention or observational research studies. However, some lifestyle factors are harder to conduct similar studies. However, there is accumulating evidence to point to thar relaxation techniques are effective in reducing stress, and by doing this likely reduces the chance of a heart attack. Sudden or intense emotional or physical stressors such as an argument or heavy physical exertion can result in vasospasm of coronary arteries or acute rupture of an atherosclerotic plaque – both of which can lead to a heart attack. Chronic stress such as home or work stress, reduced ability to control one's day to day affairs – can also increase the risk of heart attack. Relaxation techniques with research evidence to support their effectiveness include yoga and meditation (Chong et al., 2011; Harne et al., 2019). Yoga focusses on breathing regulation and stretching and regular practice is association with reduced blood pressure and cardiovascular events (Hagins et al., 2013). We all have stress and if Yoga is part of your traditional prayers and practice that is a great component of your lifestyle, but if it is not, you may consider seeking out more knowledge and begin the practice to optimize your health and stress management.

Meditation and Breathing Techniques:
Other social activities combine physical activity and tend to have a positive effect on mental health - such as a group or pair dancing, joining sports teams, or regular outdoor activities imbibing the beauty of our natural world. Social connectedness has been shown to be associated with lower chronic diseases and greater longevity. Data from the Framingham study by Nicholas Christakis has shown that social isolation and loneliness are associated with a range of negative health outcomes, including increased risk of cardiovascular disease, depression, and premature death (Christakis & Fowler, 2007; Kim et al., 2016; Rosenquist et al., 2011). The Harvard longitudinal health study showed that loneliness was as potent as cigarette smoking causing death (Cacioppo et al., 2009). Other data show after the loss of a loved one how grief and loneliness accelerate mortality. This study published in the journal "Heart" in 2016, analyzed data from more than 3.4 million people and found that those who reported feeling lonely or socially isolated had a significantly higher risk of dying prematurely than those who did not (Otto, 2016). Specifically, the study found that people who reported feeling lonely had a 26% higher risk of dying prematurely, while those who reported living alone had a 32% higher risk of dying prematurely (Otto, 2016). These findings suggest that social isolation and loneliness are important public health concerns that should be taken seriously.

What does the Ayurveda show about this: mental stress and techniques to resolve it?

The Ayurvedic body of knowledge is the holistic perspective of health that emphasizes the interconnectedness of the body and mind (Basisht, 2014). Ayurveda views stress as an imbalance of the mind and body, caused by various factors such as poor diet, lack of exercise, and emotional disturbances. Therefore, mental health and physical health cannot be siloed and treated separately. Thus, mental stressors such as anxiety, grief, or anger are treated with the same level of gravity as physical stressors (ex., exhaustion, excessive physical exercise, or injury) and environmental stressors (ex. high altitudes or exposure to intense heat) (Shree Gulabkunverba Ayurvedic Society, 2024). Ayurvedic stress management techniques aim to restore balance and promote relaxation, thereby reducing stress levels and improving overall well-being.

Ayurveda is based on the concept of the three doshas, or energies, that are believed to circulate in the body: Vata, Pitta, and Kapha. Each person is believed to have a unique combination of these doshas, which influences their physical and mental characteristics, as well as their susceptibility to certain health problems. Ayurvedic practitioners use a range of techniques to balance the doshas and promote health, including diet and nutrition, herbal medicine, massage and bodywork, yoga, meditation, and lifestyle changes. **Ayurveda emphasizes the importance of maintaining balance and harmony in all aspects of life, including diet, sleep, exercise, and emotional well-being.** Some Ayurvedic remedies for mental stress include meditation, yoga, aromatherapy, and some herbs. The first three have been popularized in western culture as well and there are many resources available. Ayurvedic herbs are also promoted and sought but these should be only used after consultation with an Ayurvedic practitioner ideally well trained as some herbs can cause unexpected reactions. Furthermore, sometimes mental illness is significant enough that conventional medicine is required with effective pharmacotherapies to treat conditions such as depression, anxiety, and psychosis.

Multiple randomized and non-randomized studies have demonstrated the effectiveness of mindfulness meditation as a strategy to reduce stress, depression, anxiety, and distress and to improve quality of life (Khoury et al., 2015).

Yoga incorporates elements of physical poses, breathing exercises and meditation, as well as lifestyle habits such as moderation in diet and abstinence from smoking and alcohol. Over the past 5 decades the health benefits of yoga have been tried and tested. Multiple randomized trials have demonstrated the effectiveness of Yoga on reducing self reported stress (subjective) and objective measures of stress including cortisol, systolic blood pressure, heart rate, heart rate variability, Yoga reduced fasting blood glucose, cholesterol and low density lipoprotein (Pascoe et al., 2017). A recent trial conducted in India by my colleague Prabhakaran showed that the practice of Yoga tended to reduce recurrent major cardiac events and improve self-reported quality of life in patients with established heart disease (Prabhakaran et al., 2020).

Isn't it ironic that these practices are South Asian in their origin, and promoted > 3000 years ago, and still apply in modern times, and require western evaluation techniques to be "proven" right?! In the next chapter these traditional practices will be reviewed, and many hold the secret to a healthy life.

REFERENCES

Anand, S. S., Islam, S., Rosengren, A., Franzosi, M. G., Steyn, K., Yusufali, A. H., Keltai, M., Diaz, R., Rangarajan, S., Yusuf, S., & on behalf of the INTERHEART Investigators. (2008). Risk factors for myocardial infarction in women and men: Insights from the INTERHEART study. European Heart Journal, 29(7), 932–940. https://doi.org/10.1093/eurheartj/ehn018

Basisht, G. (2014). Exploring insights towards definition and laws of health in Ayurveda: Global health perspective. Ayu, 35(4), 351–355. https://doi.org/10.4103/0974-8520.158975

Bulatao, R. A., Anderson, N. B., & National Research Council (US) Panel on Race, E. (2004). Stress. In Understanding Racial and Ethnic Differences in Health in Late Life: A Research Agenda. National Academies Press (US). https://www.ncbi.nlm.nih.gov/books/NBK24685/

Cacioppo, J. T., Fowler, J. H., & Christakis, N. A. (2009). Alone in the Crowd: The Structure and Spread of Loneliness in a Large Social Network. Journal of Personality and Social Psychology, 97(6), 977–991. https://doi.org/10.1037/a0016076

Chong, C. S. M., Tsunaka, M., Tsang, H. W. H., Chan, E. P., & Cheung, W. M. (2011). Effects of yoga on stress management in healthy adults: A systematic review. Alternative Therapies in Health and Medicine, 17(1), 32–38.

Christakis, N. A., & Fowler, J. H. (2007). The spread of obesity in a large social network over 32 years. The New England Journal of Medicine, 357(4), 370–379. https://doi.org/10.1056/NEJMsa066082

Connelly, D. (2021, July 22). In figures: The science of stress. The Pharmaceutical Journal. https://pharmaceutical-journal.com/article/feature/in-figures-the-science-of-stress

Czech, M. P., Tencerova, M., Pedersen, D. J., & Aouadi, M. (2013). Insulin signalling mechanisms for triacylglycerol storage. Diabetologia, 56(5), 949–964. https://doi.org/10.1007/s00125-013-2869-1

Grossman, P., Niemann, L., Schmidt, S., & Walach, H. (2004). Mindfulness-based stress reduction and health benefits: A meta-analysis. Journal of Psychosomatic Research, 57(1), 35–43. https://doi.org/10.1016/S0022-3999(03)00573-7

Hagins, M., States, R., Selfe, T., & Innes, K. (2013). Effectiveness of Yoga for Hypertension: Systematic Review and Meta-Analysis. Evidence-Based Complementary and Alternative Medicine : eCAM, 2013, 649836. https://doi.

org/10.1155/2013/649836

Harne, B. P., Tahseen, A. A., Hiwale, A. S., & Dhekekar, R. S. (2019). Survey on Om meditation: Its effects on the human body and Om meditation as a tool for stress management. Psychological Thought, 12(1). https://www.psycharchives.org/en/item/be838e6a-cac6-49e5-b57e-c29993b6637a

Herhaus, B., Ullmann, E., Chrousos, G., & Petrowski, K. (2020). High/low cortisol reactivity and food intake in people with obesity and healthy weight. Translational Psychiatry, 10(1), 1–8. https://doi.org/10.1038/s41398-020-0729-6

Ip, C. K., Rezitis, J., Qi, Y., Bajaj, N., Koller, J., Farzi, A., Shi, Y.-C., Tasan, R., Zhang, L., & Herzog, H. (2023). Critical role of lateral habenula circuits in the control of stress-induced palatable food consumption. Neuron, 111(16), 2583-2600.e6. https://doi.org/10.1016/j.neuron.2023.05.010

Khoury, B., Sharma, M., Rush, S. E., & Fournier, C. (2015). Mindfulness-based stress reduction for healthy individuals: A meta-analysis. Journal of Psychosomatic Research, 78(6), 519–528. https://doi.org/10.1016/j.jpsychores.2015.03.009

Kim, D. A., Benjamin, E. J., Fowler, J. H., & Christakis, N. A. (2016). Social connectedness is associated with fibrinogen level in a human social network. Proceedings. Biological Sciences, 283(1837), 20160958. https://doi.org/10.1098/rspb.2016.0958

Lagraauw, H. M., Kuiper, J., & Bot, I. (2015). Acute and chronic psychological stress as risk factors for cardiovascular disease: Insights gained from epidemiological, clinical and experimental studies. Brain, Behavior, and Immunity, 50, 18–30. https://doi.org/10.1016/j.bbi.2015.08.007

Li, J., Zhang, M., Loerbroks, A., Angerer, P., & Siegrist, J. (2014). Work stress and the risk of recurrent coronary heart disease events: A systematic review and meta-analysis. International Journal of Occupational Medicine and Environmental Health. https://doi.org/10.2478/s13382-014-0303-7

Marmot, M., & Brunner, E. (2005). Cohort Profile: The Whitehall II study. International Journal of Epidemiology, 34(2), 251–256. https://doi.org/10.1093/ije/dyh372

Maté, G. (2003). When the body says no: The cost of hidden stress (1st ed). A.A. Knopf Canada.

Mirza, S., Kandasamy, S., Souza, R. J. de, Wahi, G., Desai, D., Anand, S. S., & Ritvo, P. (2022). Barriers and facilitators to healthy active living in South Asian families in Canada: A thematic analysis. BMJ Open, 12(11), e060385. https://doi.org/10.1136/bmjopen-2021-060385

Otto, C. M. (2016). Heartbeat: Lonely Hearts. Heart, 102(13), 985–986. https://doi.org/10.1136/heartjnl-2016-310034

Pascoe, M. C., Thompson, D. R., & Ski, C. F. (2017). Yoga, mindfulness-based stress reduction and stress-related physiological measures: A meta-analysis. Psychoneuroendocrinology, 86, 152–168. https://doi.org/10.1016/j.psyneuen.2017.08.008

Prabhakaran, D., Chandrasekaran, A. M., Singh, K., Mohan, B., Chattopadhyay, K., Chadha, D. S., Negi, P. C., Bhat, P., Sadananda, K. S., Ajay, V. S., Singh, K., Praveen, P. A., Devarajan, R., Kondal, D., Soni, D., Mallinson, P., Manchanda, S. C., Madan, K., Hughes, A. D., ... Madappa, N. U. (2020). Yoga-Based Cardiac Rehabilitation After Acute Myocardial Infarction: A Randomized Trial. Journal of the American College of Cardiology, 75(13), 1551–1561. https://doi.org/10.1016/j.jacc.2020.01.050

Rosengren, A., Hawken, S., Ôunpuu, S., Sliwa, K., Zubaid, M., Almahmeed, W. A., Blackett, K. N., Sitthi-amorn, C., Sato, H., & Yusuf, S. (2004). Association of psychosocial risk factors with risk of acute myocardial infarction in 11 119 cases and 13 648 controls from 52 countries (the INTERHEART study): Case-control study. The Lancet, 364(9438), 953–962. https://doi.org/10.1016/S0140-6736(04)17019-0

Rosenquist, J., Fowler, J., & Christakis, N. (2011). Social network determinants of depression. Molecular Psychiatry, 16(3), 10.1038/mp.2010.13. https://doi.org/10.1038/mp.2010.13

Shree Gulabkunverba Ayurvedic Society. (2024, November 30). Charaka Samhita (English translation). Wisdom Library. https://www.wisdomlib.org/hinduism/book/charaka-samhita-english

Torres, S. J., & Nowson, C. A. (2007). Relationship between stress, eating behavior, and obesity. Nutrition, 23(11), 887–894. https://doi.org/10.1016/j.nut.2007.08.008

Vahedian-Azimi, A., & Moayed, M. S. (2019). Updating the Meta-Analysis of Perceived Stress and its Association with the Incidence of Coronary Heart Disease. International Journal of Medical Reviews, 6(4), 146–153. https://doi.org/10.30491/ijmr.2019.101968

Yusuf, S., Hawken, S., Ôunpuu, S., Dans, T., Avezum, A., Lanas, F., McQueen, M., Budaj, A., Pais, P., Varigos, J., & Lisheng, L. (2004). Effect of potentially modifiable risk factors associated with myocardial infarction in 52 countries (the INTERHEART study): Case-control study. The Lancet, 364(9438), 937–952. https://doi.org/10.1016/S0140-6736(04)17018-9

Chapter 7

Medications can also be used to treat risk factors, and are very effective

Why are people so resistant to take prescription medications?

In my experience seeing patients referred with single or multiple risk factors but who have NOT had a serious clinical event such as a heart attack are extremely RESISTANT to start medications to treat the risk factors and to PREVENT such serious clinical events. Let's explore what underlies this resistance?

> **When do I need to consider medications or even surgery?**
> (High risk primary and secondary prevention)

- **Cholesterol lowering**
- Weight Loss – medications, surgery
(GLP-1's "Wegovy", Liposuction, Bariatric surgery)
- **Diabetes medications**
- **Heart Disease**
(Once I have heart disease do I take these for life?)
- **What about my risks for Stroke and Cancer?**

First off, I understand this feeling on a personal level as I also am a minimalist when it comes to having medical tests and taking exogenous substances, if I don't have to. I take minimal pain medications or other such medications with mild illness or after surgery. I also have personal experience of caring for my elderly parents, my physician Mother did not like to take prescription medications either, and the only ones she took seriously were her medications related to breast cancer, and her blood pressure medication because she did not want to suffer a stroke. My Father, as general surgeon who was precise and meticulous in his day-to-day work, kept a detailed list, a dosette, and in his final years had a blister package to be sure he followed doctor's orders to a tee, and often recorded his blood pressure and checked off a list to indicate he had taken his daily medications. My patients vary widely between requiring multiple conversations over the span of a year to help them decide if they will start a medication to prevent cardiovascular disease, to being very adherent and observant, and who bring in new information they have read to ensure they are being maximally treated with medications to prevent CVD.

The top reasons people do not want to take a prescription medication:

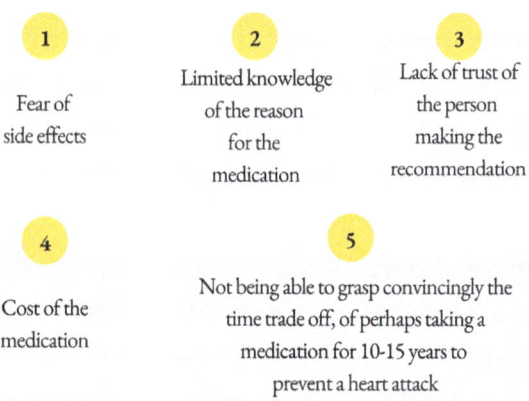

1 Fear of side effects

2 Limited knowledge of the reason for the medication

3 Lack of trust of the person making the recommendation

4 Cost of the medication

5 Not being able to grasp convincingly the time trade off, of perhaps taking a medication for 10-15 years to prevent a heart attack

If an ounce of prevention equals a pound of cure, why aren't all patients interested or motivated to take prescription medications?

Surveys of North Americans indicate that the most **trusted** professionals include nurses and doctors. Nurses and doctors who build trust by spending more time with their patients do succeed more often in shifting patient's beliefs from being skeptical, to becoming believers in the value of the **information** provided. Their recommendations are informed by the evidence from randomized trials, combined with the years of clinical experience, and this experience is far superior to the advice of "Dr Google" which is so common today. During the COVID-19 pandemic we surveyed South Asians in the Greater Toronto Area and asked them what their most trusted sources of information were, and they endorsed: 1) health care professionals, 2) public health professionals, and 3) mainstream newspapers and television (Anand et al., 2022). The source of information and trust in who is providing the information – are crucial components of the decision-making process, but not the only components.

Beginning to take a prescription medication is beginning a commitment to prevent a health problem like a heart attack or stroke in the future. This is like taking one's car into the auto shop to have a regular check-up and servicing to prevent an unexpected failure in the braking system or transmission – with one key difference. While brake failure can result in death, a transmission failure usually wont, but it can be financially very costly. In Canada with a universal health care plan, to see a physician isn't **costly**, however the absence of a universal pharmacare plan can be, especially for the more expensive medications which are not off patent protection. However low-cost effective medications exist to treat most risk factors for cholesterol lowering, blood pressure lowering, and diabetes. This covers ¾'s of the risk factors that need treatment. However, absence of a drug plan through employment insurance can pose a barrier for more recently patented diabetes, weight loss, cholesterol lowering, and Lp(a) lowering medications.

Apart from knowledge, trust, and cost, a remaining barrier for patient's who have "silent risk factors" like elevated cholesterol, mild elevations in blood sugar and blood pressure, who cannot **"feel the risk"** in contrast to a patient who had to call 911 for chest pain, gone through the Emergency Room Department, undergone a coronary angiogram, and ended up in the coronary care unit. As I often say to my patients, you could take this prevention medication NOW to treat your risk factors to prevent needing to go to hospital, or not taking the medications and face the possibility of ending up unexpectedly in hospital, and being placed on **4 to 5 new medications all at once**. **Time trade-off** is a concept often used in health care economics to understand how people value different health states over time. These studies seek to understand how much time in perfect health people are willing to trade off to avoid potential side effects or risks associated with medication use. The decisions are influenced by many factors including a person's unconscious biases, life experiences, and cultural beliefs. However, some factors may be more consistently influential for certain individuals or populations. Within the South Asian diaspora, spiritual beliefs may also play a role. For example, the concept of Belief in **Kismet** often reflects a fatalistic outlook, where individuals may attribute events to destiny or divine will. Amongst others, cultural beliefs in **karma**, which is the concept of cause and effect, may influence the perception that lifestyle choices and actions play a significant role in health outcomes. Individuals might prioritize lifestyle modifications as a means of influencing their health rather than relying solely on medications.

It is then no surprise given how many factors go into influencing a decision to take a prescription medication that the World Health Organization (WHO) reports that **only 50% of all patients given a prescription**, actually take the medication on a consistent basis (Sabaté, 2003). If each patient had a "post prescription" therapist or health coach this percentage could increase. Research supporting the effectiveness of health coaching is growing, particularly in areas like weight management, diabetes prevention, and overall well-being (Kivelä et al., 2014). Where something like this has been evaluated, adherence to a lifestyle program or medication program with regular interaction of health coach or personal trainer increases by two-fold. **Support groups** such as a Health Network or a social network that emphasizes health could in fact be very effective, as could discussion and support from a local pharmacist, local faith-based community, or health charities such as the American Heart Association or Heart and Stroke Foundation. Your reading of this book makes you thus very knowledgeable and perhaps you can set into motion in your own sphere of influence, the provision of information, trust, and access to support the South Asian community in Heart Health.

All recommendations here have been proven to be effective and safe in randomized controlled trials. This is the highest level of evidence in clinical research and is far higher than 'taking advice' from your neighbour, reading about new fad on the internet, watching youtube, or from your local health food store. Of course, the decision to take prescription medication should be made together with your doctor. These medications include:

Glucose-lowering medications

There are 8 classes of medications your doctors can choose from, all of them have indications that can be tailored to your specific set of risk factors.

1. Metformin in patients with pre-diabetes, and type 2 diabetes and is usually first line.

2. SGLT-2 inhibitors such as empaglaflozin or jiardiance lower glucose, reduce cardiovascular events, and bring about some weight loss.

3. GLP-1 receptor agonists such as liraglutide and semaglutide (Ozempic) - these are injectable agents, reduce blood glucose and yield significant weight loss

4. DPP-4 inhibitors (inhibit the enzyme that breakdown GLP-i1) thereby creating a similar effect of GLP-1agonists. Examples include sitagliptin or Januvia.

5. Alpha-glucosidase or Acarbose.

6. Secreatogogues such as glyburide.

7. Thiazidenolones including pio and rosiglitozine.

8. Insulin – injectable.

Medication Class Name	Example Medications	Trade Names
Biguanides	Metformin	Glucophage, Fortamet, Riomet
Sulfonylureas	Glipizide, Glyburide	Glucotrol, DiaBeta, Micronase
Meglitinides	Repaglinide, Nateglinide	Prandin, Starlix
Dipeptidyl Peptidase-4 Inhibitors (DPP-4 Inhibitors)	Sitagliptin, Saxagliptin	Januvia, Onglyza
Thiazolidinediones	Pioglitazone, Rosiglitazone	Actos, Avandia
Alpha-glucosidase Inhibitors	Acarbose, Miglitol	Precose, Glyset
Sodium-Glucose Cotransporter-2 (SGLT-2) Inhibitors	Canagliflozin, Dapagliflozin	Invokana, Farxiga
GLP-1 Receptor Agonists	Exenatide, Liraglutide	Byetta, Victoza
Insulin	Regular insulin, Insulin glargine	Humulin, Novolin, Lantus, Levemir

Cholesterol-lowering medications

As indicated in earlier chapters there is a substantial body of clinical trial evidence providing support for LDL reduction with statins in reducing cardiovascular events. The Cholesterol lowering trialists collaboration show through a meta-analysis of trials that a 1 mmol/L reduction in LDL is associated with a 20% reduction in major cardiovascular events (Baigent et al., 2005).

1. Statin medications which are very effective and well tolerated.
2. Ezetimibe.
3. PCSK-9 inhibitors.
4. Highly purified fish oil.
5. Fibrates.

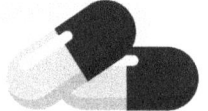

Medication Class	Example Medications	Trade Names
Statins	Atorvastatin, Simvastatin, Rosuvastatin	Lipitor, Zocor, Crestor
Ezetimibe (Cholesterol Absorption Inhibitor)	Ezetimibe	Zetia
Bile Acid Sequestrants	Cholestyramine, Colesevelam, Colestipol	Questran, Welchol, Colestid
PCSK9 Inhibitors	Alirocumab, Evolocumab	Praluent, Repatha
Fibrates	Gemfibrozil, Fenofibrate	Lopid, Tricor, Fenoglide
Niacin (Nicotinic Acid)	Niacin	Niaspan
Highly Purified Fish Oil		Vascepa

Blood Pressure-lowering agents

If you have high blood pressure, then blood pressure-lowering medications are widely available, and very effective.

1 ACE inhibitors or ARBs.

2 Diuretics.

3 Beta-Blockers.

4 Calcium channel blockers.

5 Mineralocorticoids.

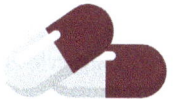

Medication Class	Example Medications	Trade Names
ACE Inhibitors	Enalapril, Lisinopril	Vasotec, Prinivil, Zestril
	Losartan, Valsartan	Cozaar, Diovan
Diuretics	Hydrochlorothiazide (HCTZ)	Microzide, HydroDIU-RIL
	Furosemide	Lasix
Beta-Blockers	Metoprolol, Atenolol	Lopressor, Tenormin
	Propranolol	Inderal
Calcium Channel Blockers	Amlodipine, Nifedipine	Norvasc, Procardia
	Diltiazem	Cardizem
Mineralocorticoids	Spironolactone	Aldactone

Therapeutic agents for weight loss:
There are increasing options to bring about weight loss using medications. Most people would have heard of "Ozempic" or "Wegovy" otherwise known as semaglutide, a GLP-1 agonist. This injectable medication, through its promotion of GLP-1, leads to a reduced desire to eat food,

thereby resulting in weight loss with long-term use (15% weight loss) and among diabetics reduces blood glucose (HbA1c by 2%), and LDL cholesterol. This medication is effective as proven in randomized controlled trials, and side effects are more common when higher doses are used, and can include diarrhea, nausea, and vomiting (Yao et al., 2024).

Bariatric surgery is a type of surgical procedure that is designed to help people who are severely overweight or obese lose weight. The procedure involves reducing the size of the stomach, which helps to limit the amount of food a person can eat, and in some cases, also changes how the body absorbs nutrients. Bariatric surgery results in weight reduction of approximately 25 to 30% at 1 to 2 years (van Rijswijk et al., 2021).

Deciding what weight loss approaches are best for you, should be made together with your physician, and tailored to your metabolic needs and other health and lifestyle factors.

Medication Class	Example Medications	Trade Names
Orlistat (Lipase Inhibitor)	Orlistat	Xenical, Alli
Phentermine (Sympathomimetic Amine)	Phentermine	Adipex-P, Lomaira
GLP-1 Receptor Agonists	Liraglutide, Semaglutide	Saxenda, Ozempic
Naltrexone and Bupropion (Combination)	Naltrexone/Bupropion	Contrave

Other Medications: What about aspirin, my patient's report hearing from the news media and friends that it is good to keep a bottle of aspirin in the house in case someone has signs of a heart attack, and ask "is aspirin something I should take daily?"

Aspirin inhibits the production and function of platelets, components of the blood that makes it sticky. If a patient takes aspirin, it decreases the risk of a blood clot forming in a critical artery and thereby can reduce the chance of a serious heart attack. However, the downside is that bleeding can be caused by regular aspirin use. Therefore, it is important to discuss with your physician who can help you weight the benefits versus the risks of taking a regular aspirin.

Will taking medications to prevent CV disease also help to prevent stroke and cancer?

Although physicians and researchers often specialize in treating one disease, patients don't think this way, of course we all fear getting cancer – because although for some cancers there are cures, for the most common cancers, we have seen loved one, struggle through surgery, radiation, and chemotherapy which is trying on the body, and impairs quality and often quantity of life. Most people are not as fearful of having a heart attack but remain fearful about having a stroke or limb amputation. It is very informative to see in the table below that as an individual's trying to prevent one condition, the health improvements you make will likely reduce your chances of having the other conditions. Health active living with a high diet quality, minimal excessive fat accumulation, low to no alcohol intake, avoidance of tobacco products, will reduce your risk of some cancers.

Risk Factor	**Heart Attack**	**Stroke**	**Cancer**
Age	Increased risk with age	Increased risk with age	Increased risk with age
Tobacco Use	✓	✓	✓
Diet and Nutrition	✓	✓	✓
Physical Inactivity	✓	✓	✓
Obesity	✓	✓	✓
Hypertension	✓	✓	Not common
Diabetes	✓	✓	Some types
Alcohol Consumption	Moderate to excessive	Moderate to excessive	Moderate to excessive
Genetics/Family History	✓	✓	Some types
Chronic Inflammation	✓	✓	✓
Environmental Exposures e.g. Air Pollution	✓	✓	✓

Will I have to take these medications for life?

This is a question I often hear from people I help with their health. After I share information and they agree that they need medicine, they ask this question. The answer is, "It depends."

For people with risk factors who haven't had a serious event like a heart attack or stroke—especially if they also have things like too much body fat or not-so-healthy eating habits—I might suggest starting the medicine. Then, we agree to keep an eye on their health habits and how their risk factors are doing over time.

For example, if someone really wants to improve their diet and do more physical activities, and they succeed in losing extra body fat, their blood pressure, cholesterol, and blood sugar could get better. So, watching and checking regularly is a good way to go. This is different than for someone with genetics that makes their cholesterol high; no matter how much they change their lifestyle, their risk stays high.

Now, for people who already had a heart attack or stroke, most of the medicines they are placed on should be continued life-long. But, it still depends on each person. If someone loses a lot of weight, their blood pressure and blood sugar might drop, and then we may need to rethink some of the medicines. On the other hand, some might still have issues despite taking the best medicines, so we might need to change doses or add more medicines.

Summary:
The good news is that a healthy active living lifestyle pattern will optimize your chances for chronic disease free health, and when required there are many treatments that can be delivered to prevent heart disease in South Asians - if risk factors are identified and modified early. However, for those of us who prefer to try and alter components of how we live to prevent heart disease for ourselves and our children, these lifestyle changes need to begin in youth by hardwiring certain lifestyle features into daily living routines. It is very difficult to successfully make these changes once they have become routine, not impossible, but very difficult. Sometimes when risk factors for CVD are identified by your physician, they will recommend a medication should be initiated to reduce your risk. Many people are reluctant to use medications, however there is a strong clinical trials evidence base to treat common CV risk factors, and addressing them early is like investing in an RRSP or compounding interest program, to prevent CV disease, "no wealth without health" as they say.

REFERENCES

Anand, S. S., Arnold, C., Bangdiwala, S. I., Bolotin, S., Bowdish, D., Chanchlani, R., Souza, R. J. de, Desai, D., Kandasamy, S., Khan, F., Khan, Z., Langlois, M.-A., Limbachia, J., Lear, S. A., Loeb, M., Loh, L., Manoharan, B., Nakka, K., Pelchat, M., … Wahi, G. (2022). Seropositivity and risk factors for SARS-CoV-2 infection in a South Asian community in Ontario: A cross-sectional analysis of a prospective cohort study. Canadian Medical Association Open Access Journal, 10(3), E599–E609. https://doi.org/10.9778/cmajo.20220031

Baigent, C., Keech, A., Kearney, P. M., Blackwell, L., Buck, G., Pollicino, C., Kirby, A., Sourjina, T., Peto, R., Collins, R., Simes, R., & Cholesterol Treatment Trialists' (CTT) Collaborators. (2005). Efficacy and safety of cholesterol-lowering treatment: Prospective meta-analysis of data from 90,056 participants in 14 randomised trials of statins. Lancet (London, England), 366(9493), 1267–1278. https://doi.org/10.1016/S0140-6736(05)67394-1

Kivelä, K., Elo, S., Kyngäs, H., & Kääriäinen, M. (2014). The effects of health coaching on adult patients with chronic diseases: A systematic review. Patient Education and Counseling, 97(2), 147–157. https://doi.org/10.1016/j.pec.2014.07.026

Sabaté, E. (Ed.). (2003). Adherence to long-term therapies: Evidence for action. World Health Organization.

van Rijswijk, A.-S., van Olst, N., Schats, W., van der Peet, D. L., & van de Laar, A. W. (2021). What Is Weight Loss After Bariatric Surgery Expressed in Percentage Total Weight Loss (%TWL)? A Systematic Review. Obesity Surgery, 31(8), 3833–3847. https://doi.org/10.1007/s11695-021-05394-x

Yao, H., Zhang, A., Li, D., Wu, Y., Wang, C.-Z., Wan, J.-Y., & Yuan, C.-S. (2024). Comparative effectiveness of GLP-1 receptor agonists on glycaemic control, body weight, and lipid profile for type 2 diabetes: Systematic review and network meta-analysis. BMJ, 384, e076410. https://doi.org/10.1136/bmj-2023-076410

Chapter 8

What is the role of Ayurvedic medicine?

On his second appointment, Rajinder's mother accompanied him to the clinic. When I asked Rajinder about his progress in making some changes to his dietary intake and physical activity, as he started speaking, I noticed his mother was quietly shaking her head in disagreement. I asked her for her opinion on how things were going. She told me that her son only needed to listen to her teachings and follow her practice of Ayurvedic medicine to remain healthy. In this ancient practice individuals are classified by their DOSHAs, and the combinations of Doshas led to classification by Prakriti:

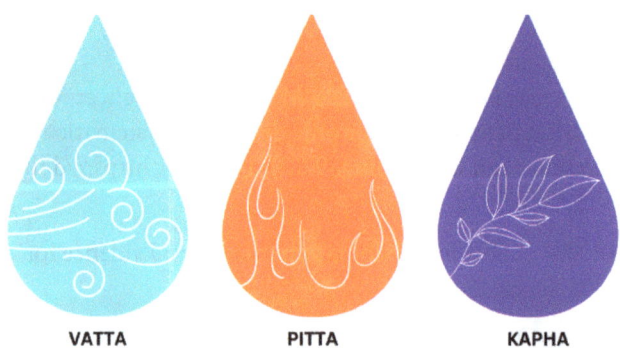

VATTA   **PITTA**   **KAPHA**

VATTA, PITTA and KAPHA, each with a certain set of attributes, high energy to lower energy, and aligned with the DOSHAs were recommended foods, types of exercise, and sleep patterns to align with optimal health and well-being. These constitutional types are unique to different individuals based on the attributes of their personality. When these doshas are in equilibrium, the body achieves perfect health and harmony. An imbalance or degradation of doshas increases morbidity of various diseases.

Ayurveda has a deep-rooted cultural and historical significance in India, and a significant proportion of India's population incorporates Ayurvedic principles into their daily lives. The use of Ayurveda varies across different regions, communities, and individuals. The importance of sleep cannot be understated in the Ayurveda. Sleep is considered to be integral to our physiology and is a basic, yet essential, instinct in life (Prajapati & Paliwal, 2019; Telles, Sharma, et al., 2015). Early descriptions of sleep and sleep disorders trace back to 100 BC - 900 AD in the Sushruta Samhita. Subsequent mentions occur in the Charaka Samhita (300-500 AD) and Vagbatta (700 AD). The general sentiment in the scripture is that an adequate amount of sleep is needed for maintaining good health. Ayurvedic medicine does not view diet, psychology, or exercise in silos, but instead takes a holistic perspective on human health and wellbeing such that these factors are considered when considering the topic of sleep. It is amazing to read the ancient wisdom and its emphasis on the interconnection between the mind and body, and the consideration of mental stresses being as substantial as physical stresses. Proper sleep cycles, diet (e.g., avoid sweet, food as medicine etc....), and tailoring the type and intensity of exercise to the Dosha, and warning about the risk of over exertion, how to approach obesity using herbal medicine, mindfulness, diet and lifestyle along with stress management. Table 1 displays the characteristics of each Ayruvedic category across a range of health behaviours.

Western scientific evidence and the way that it is validated through randomized controlled trials for example, feature predominantly in this book as these are the methods by which I am trained, and the type of research I have conducted. However, there is research being conducted predominantly in India to validate Ayurvedic practices using similar methods. For example, the Central Council for Research in Ayurvedic Sciences (CCRAS), serves as the research body in Ayurveda in India. CCRAS operates under the Ministry of Ayurveda, Yoga & Naturopathy, Unani, Siddha, and Homoeopathy (AYUSH) run by the Government of India. AYUSH recommendations to prevent heart disease are largely consistent with the ones in this book. From their website you will see alignment in types of foods, maintaining a healthy waist circumference, having adequate sleep, stress reduction, using salt in moderation, and minimizing sugar consumption (Ministry of Ayush, n.d.).

	VATA (air + space)	**PITTA** (fire + water)	**KAPHA** (water + earth)
Sleep Cycle	Interrupted sleep, insomnia, daytime restlessness	Restlessness	Tendency to oversleep, feeling sluggish
Diet	Variable appetite, tendency to forget meals, sensitive digestive patterns leading to bloating and constipation. Gravitate to bitter, dried, and cold foods.	Acid reflux, heartburn, diarrhea, frequent hunger pangs and excessive thirst, inflammatory responses. Gravitate to spicy and heavy foods. Often crave intense and flavorful foods.	Imbalances such as weight gain, lethargy, and congestion. Gravitate to "comfort foods" that can exacerbate their natural tendencies of heaviness, coldness, and sluggishness such as heavy, sugary, fatty and/or processed foods.
Exercise type	Flexible, and free flowing movements like cycling, running, or yoga.	Team sports, tendency to go too hard.	Any movement is beneficial as long as it increases body temperature.
Obesity-holistic	Underweight or thin frame, fast metabolism, prone to feeling cold.	Good metabolism, tendency to overheat	Slow metabolism, prone to weight gain.
Stress management	Easily excitable or overwhelmed, sensitive, experiences loneliness.	Mood swings, difficulty being patient, aggressive.	Stable, reserved, patient, lack of motivation, prone to depression.

Table 1: Characteristics of Aryuvedic Categories Across Health Behaviors (Arora et al., 2003; Banerjee et al., 2015; Choudhury et al., 2018; Davidson, 2020; Payyappallimana & Venkatasubramanian, 2016; Telles, Pathak, et al., 2015)

By now you must have read common themes in this book chronicling Rajinder and Farah's journey toward improved cardiac health. Healthy active living characterized by consuming whole foods cooked at home in moderation preventing the slow creep of 1 pound of weight per year from age 20 years. Daily exercise though walking and light weight resistance training or moderate aerobic exercise through tennis, jogging, basketball are alternatives. If exercise is not part of your tradition, personal trainers are proven to work! If you can afford one, add them to your healthy active living list of priorities. Remember even if you go to the gym, sitting all day long at work or at home, independently contribute to cardio-metabolic derangements. Consider getting a standing desk, standing up and walk around every 2 hours while at work, and hold 'walking meetings'.

For Farah, she receives endless advice from her grandmother and mother about how to live a healthy life, but she finds it difficult to prioritize her health while she holds down a full-time job and raises her three daughters. In general, the Ayurvedic practices she is recommended to follow are aligned with clinic advice for healthy active living.

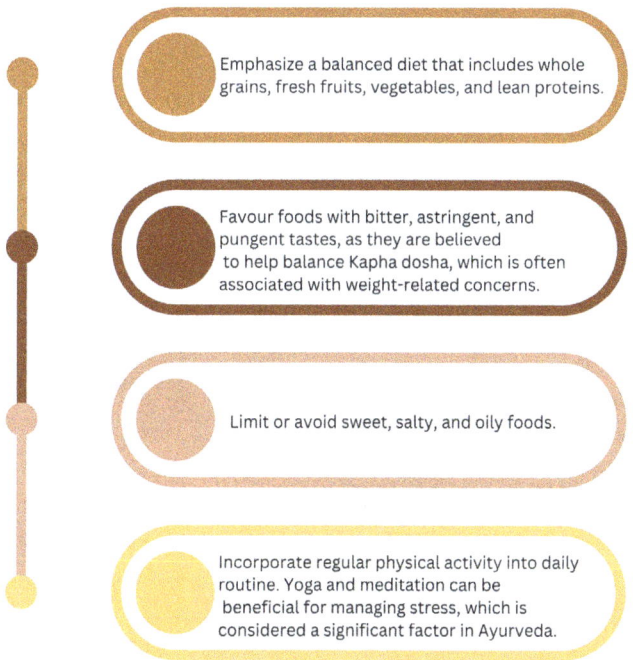

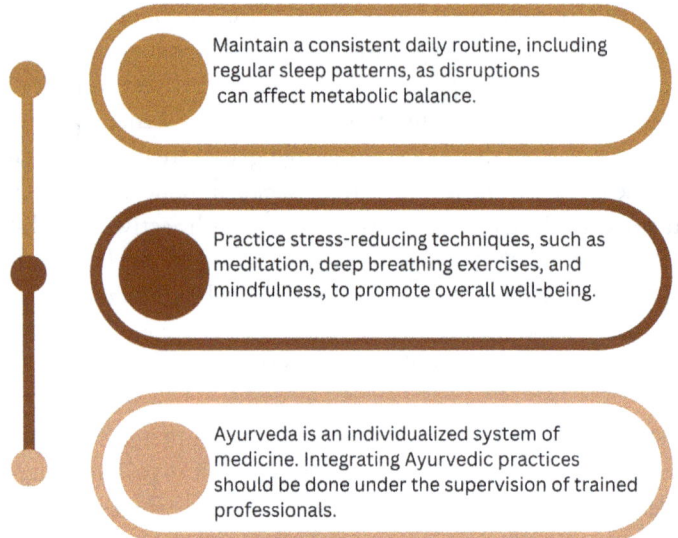

Her grandmother's advice was probably sound – she (and possibly you!) need to remember to stay in balance of mind and body and keep time each day to do so through meditation, prayer, and yoga.

Finally, if you do develop CV risk factors like abdominal obesity, elevated cholesterol, elevated glucose, or blood pressure, try and be open to the medication(s) your doctor prescribes to aid you in returning these risk factors to normal, in order to lower your risk of cardiovascular disease. They may not be needed life-long if you have not had a heart attack or stroke, they could be used short term while you rebalance your life habits. Integrating Ayurveda together with western based medicine is likely a winning combination for preventive health. Once you have overcome these risk factors and health challenges, and reached a stable lifestyle pattern with no untreated risk factors, be sure to share your wisdom and experience with those around you.

Tips for Getting Started with Exercise

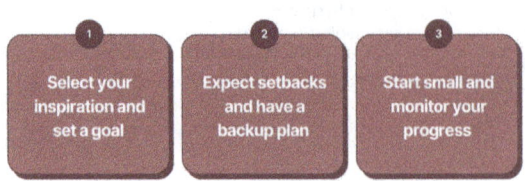

REFERENCES

Arora, D., Kumar, M., Dubey, S. D., & Baapat, S. K. (2003). Stress-Management: Leads from Ayurveda. Ancient Science of Life, 23(1), 8–15.

Banerjee, S., Debnath, P., & Debnath, P. K. (2015). Ayurnutrigenomics: Ayurveda-inspired personalized nutrition from inception to evidence. Journal of Traditional and Complementary Medicine, 5(4), 228–233. https://doi.org/10.1016/j.jtcme.2014.12.009

Choudhury, B., Kumar, V., & Basumatary, D. (2018). Management of Sthaulya (Obesity) Through Ayruveda and Yoga. 7, 356–367. https://doi.org/10.20959/wjpr201817-13302

Davidson, K. (2020, August 5). What Are the Ayurveda Doshas? Vata, Kapha, and Pitta Explained. Healthline. https://www.healthline.com/nutrition/vata-dosha-pitta-dosha-kapha-dosha

Ministry of Ayush. Care for your Heart; It will care for you too. (n.d.). Ministry of Ayush. Retrieved January 17, 2024, from https://ayushnext.ayush.gov.in/detail/post/care-for-your-heart-it-will-care-for-you-too

Payyappallimana, U., & Venkatasubramanian, P. (2016). Exploring Ayurvedic Knowledge on Food and Health for Providing Innovative Solutions to Contemporary Healthcare. Frontiers in Public Health, 4, 57. https://doi.org/10.3389/fpubh.2016.00057

Prajapati, S., & Paliwal, M. (2019). Significance of Sleep: Ayurvedic Perspective. International Journal of Health Sciences and Research, 9(1), 240–245.

Telles, S., Pathak, S., Kumar, A., Mishra, P., & Balkrishna, A. (2015). Ayurvedic Doshas as Predictors of Sleep Quality. Medical Science Monitor : International Medical Journal of Experimental and Clinical Research, 21, 1421–1427. https://doi.org/10.12659/MSM.893302

Telles, S., Sharma, S. K., Yadav, A., & Balkrishna, A. (2015). Ayurveda for Healthy Aging and Health-Related Conditions. In H. Lavretsky, M. Sajatovic, & C. Reynolds III (Eds.), Complementary and Integrative Therapies for Mental Health and Aging. Oxford University Press. https://doi.org/10.1093/med/9780199380862.003.0011

ADDITIONAL REFERENCES

Acharya, Y. (2011). Charaka Samhita with Ayurveda Deepika Teekha of Chakrapani Dutta (Reprint). Choukhambha Sanskrit Sansthan.

Basisht, G. (2014). Exploring insights towards definition and laws of health in Ayurveda: Global health perspective. Ayu, 35(4), 351–355. https://doi.org/10.4103/0974-8520.158975

Choudhary, D., Bhattacharyya, S., & Joshi, K. (2017). Body Weight Management in Adults Under Chronic Stress Through Treatment With Ashwagandha Root Extract: A Double-Blind, Randomized, Placebo-Controlled Trial. Journal of Evidence-Based Complementary & Alternative Medicine, 22(1), 96–106. https://doi.org/10.1177/2156587216641830

Joshi, V. K., & Joshi, A. (2021). Rational use of Ashwagandha in Ayurveda (Traditional Indian Medicine) for health and healing. Journal of Ethnopharmacology, 276, 114101. https://doi.org/10.1016/j.jep.2021.114101

Krishnamurthy, K. (208 C.E.). Bhela Samhitha. Chaukhambha Visvabharat.

Padakara, H. (2005). Ashtanga Hridaya with Sarvanga Sundari Commentry by Arunadatta and Ayurveda Rasayana of Hemadri (9th ed.). Krishnadas Academy.

Shaikh, J. G., & Deshmukh, S. G. (2020). Vishada (Depression) in Ayurveda: A Literary Review. International Journal of Ayurveda, 0, Article 0.

Sharma, H., Chandola, H. m., Singh, G., & Basisht, G. (2007). Utilization of Ayurveda in Health Care: An Approach for Prevention, Health Promotion, and Treatment of Disease. Part 2—Ayurveda in Primary Health Care. The Journal of Alternative and Complementary Medicine, 13(10), 1135–1150. https://doi.org/10.1089/acm.2007.7017-B

Sharma, S. (2008). Astanga Sangraha with Sasilekha Commentary by Indu (2nd ed.). Chowkhamba Sanskrit Series Office.

Toolika, E., Narayana, P., & Shetty, S. K. (2013). A Review on Ayurvedic Management of Primary Insomnia. 1(4).

Trikamji, J. (1997). Sushrutha Samhita with Nibandha Sangraha commentary of Sri Dalhanacharya (6th ed.). Chaukhamba Orientalia.

Tubaki, B. R., Chandake, S., & Sarhyal, A. (2021). Ayurveda management of Major Depressive Disorder: A case study. Journal of Ayurveda and Integrative Medicine, 12(2), 378–383. https://doi.org/10.1016/j.jaim.2021.03.012

Vaidya, A. D. B., Vaidya, R. A., Joshi, B. A., & Nabar, and N. S. (2003). Obesity (Medoroga) in Ayurveda. In Scientific Basis for Ayurvedic Therapies. Routledge.

Ven Murthy, M. R., Ranjekar, P. K., Ramassamy, C., & Deshpande, M. (2010). Scientific basis for the use of Indian ayurvedic medicinal plants in the treatment of neurodegenerative disorders: Ashwagandha. Central Nervous System Agents in Medicinal Chemistry, 10(3), 238–246. https://doi.org/10.2174/1871524911006030238

Chapter 9
Putting it all together

I have presented a lot of information which is no doubt getting your wheels turning, some of you may have already developed risk factors like diabetes, others may have, to their surprise, developed heart disease, and yet others are worried because they have seen a family member develop cardiovascular disease.

However – healthy active living improves many aspects of health and can lead you to reduce your need for medications, improve your well-being, and add to your longevity!

> First let me reassure you it is never too late to begin adopting a healthy active living program – of course, the earlier in life – the better because such a program may prevent risk factors and/or heart disease.

One important area for all of us to embed within our healthy active living programs is to ensure **we receive satisfactory amounts of sleep.** There is growing evidence that sleep quality and adequate duration are important for long-term health. Too little and too much sleep appears to be associated with adverse health outcomes like heart disease. A recent study of 74 studies showed that 7-8 hours of sleep per night appears to be the "sweet spot" for cardiovascular health (Kwok et al., 2018). It has also been shown that interrupted sleep, such as shift work has adverse metabolic consequences, altering our finely balanced stress and appetite hormones, which may cause us to overeat, and are associated with weight gain (Dutheil et al., 2020).

How did Raj and Farah fare following this program of advice?

Recall that Raj, at age 40 years was referred to me because he was found to have high cholesterol. My assessment also revealed that since moving to Canada he had gained weight and his waist circumference was now 100 cm, well above the cut off for a South Asian man, and this was reflected in his slightly elevated marker of long-term blood sugar HbA1C%. Adding to his risk he had a strong family history of early heart attack and had a marker of genetic risk called Lp(a) measured in his blood.

Luckily through this assessment and his desire to be there for his young children as they grew, and not to suffer the same fate as his father, Raj took our advice of reducing his carbohydrate intake significantly and ensuring that he walked 10,000 steps per day. After his wife attended a clinic appointment and I explained the SAHARA diet program in-depth, she took it upon herself to ensure the "food supply" in the house, and that the foods she cooked aligned with the low carb higher fibre SAHARA diet. While Raj has worked on these lifestyle features, I initiated a cholesterol lowering medication called a "statin" at low dose, and within 3 months, his non-HDL cholesterol was lowered to the primary prevention target of < 2.66 mmol/L, and with 5 pounds of weight loss, his waist circumference was reduced to 96 cm - still above the goal of 90 cm, but heading in the right direction. For follow-up, pleased that he was making progress, we planned for a repeat assessment one year after his first visit, to reassess his waist circumference, cholesterol, and blood sugar. He asked if his Lp(a) should be repeated, but because this is genetically lipoprotein and doesn't change over time, we did not plan for this. He was interested to learn more about future new therapies to reduce Lp(a) which are undergoing testing at the present time. The annual clinic appointment is a good way to assess an individual's adherence to the healthy active lifestyle program that we outlined for them, and adherence to medications. As mentioned in the previous chapters however, people are at different stages in their intent and readiness to change (Anand et al., 2016; Prochaska et al., 1992). When we assessed in the SAHARA trial amongst South Asians in Canada in whom the average risk score was in the moderate CV risk range, 72% of participants indicated to us they were **in the action or maintenance stage** to improve their diet quality, and 65% of participants indicated they were **in action or maintenance** to improve their physical activity levels.

As you can see below in the Table 1 - most of the participants in the SAHARA trial were already trying to take action on eating a health balanced diet, yet inspite of this - this group had a substantial mountain to climb as their mean baseline INTERHEART risk score was 13.3 indicating a moderate risk of future CV disease. (Anand et al., 2016).

Stage of change	Readiness Category	Examples of Motivational Statements – Healthy Eating	Proportion in the Adult SAHARA Population N=343
Precontemplation	Not Ready	"I don't really see any need to change my diet right now." "I don't think my eating habits are a problem."	7% (n=24)
Contemplation	Thinking About Change	"I've been considering eating healthier lately." "I can see how my diet might be affecting my health."	9.6% (n=33)
Preparation	Getting Ready	"I've started reading about healthy eating." "I'm planning to buy more fruits and vegetables next time I shop."	11.7% (n=40)
Action	Taking Steps	"I've started cooking more meals at home." "I've been trying out new recipes with healthier ingredients."	16.6% (n=57)
Maintenance	Sustaining Changes	"I've been consistently eating a balanced diet for the past few months." "I've found ways to make healthy eating a regular part of my routine."	55.1% (n=189)

Table 1: Readiness to Change Cardiovascular Health in the SAHARA Population Part 1 (Anand et al., 2016)

For exercising, among the SAHARA cohort, 65% reported already doing or maintaining exercise 3 x/week, this was slightly lower than the healthy eating action and maintenance, although more participants were in preparing stages for exercise 3 x per week, than were preparing for healthy eating.

For Farah, being 30 pounds above her ideal weight (which she accumulated 10 years after she finished having children) and 15 cm above her ideal waist circumference, she was on the brink of having type 2 diabetes. My advice for her included consuming a balanced high quality foods diet, (dropping the sugary beverages, simple sugars, quick carbs like bread, rice, and pasta), performing a regular exercise program, as the mainstay of her management. When she returned to be reassessed 6 months later - progress was minimal. She tried her best initially and lost 5 pounds, but with one of her children struggling at school, and her husband being constantly away for work – she regained this soon afterwards. I once again described her risk of diabetes and associated cardiovascular disease - she understood – said she would try again, and we agreed to recheck her blood work. Unfortunately, I observed she had now developed a higher HbA1C% and an elevated ALT indicating she likely had fatty liver. We spoke on the phone and wanted to try once more – this time with an app called NoomTM and a personal trainer at the gym. You agreed to wait for another 6 months to recheck her blood work – in the meantime you would also assess her liver with an ultrasound and a measure of atherosclerosis in her carotid arteries or "sludge in her pipes". When she returned in 6 months with all of her blood work and tests – the summary showed little change in her waist circumference, and now she had clear evidence of diabetes, fatty liver and more than expected atherosclerosis in her carotid arteries. We then agreed that starting a GLP-1 agonist medication called Ozempic would be a reasonable next step.

Sometimes people are confused by all the health advice on the internet Instagram or Tik Tok, what they hear from friends and relatives, and sometimes even from their physicians. Based on 25 years of research what is clear to me is that for South Asian heart health the following practices should be adopted: **Consuming a balanced low carbohydrate diet is more beneficial for your health especially fat loss than not making any dietary changes and trying only exercise to achieve weight loss. Individuals who can do both healthy eating and exercise can make real and long-lasting dietary changes to bring about fat loss AND have the most success in losing fat where it counts.** Finally, for South Asians, despite everything you have heard and believed and still hear today

– a low carbohydrate diet is more beneficial than an exercise-based program without making any changes in your diet. You might have a gym which you love to attend – so carry on with that, but if gym memberships have never worked out for your lifestyle, no worries, walking is free!

What can I do now to prevent heart disease?

- Daily walking aiming for 10,000 steps per day.
- Reduce packaged "fast" or ultra-processed foods, especially added sugar.
- Lower carbohydrate food intake; aim for a 10 carbohydrate : 1 gram of fibre ratio when reading package labels.
- Get an adequate amount of sleep.
- Lifelong health starts from childhood, so counsel your family members and lead by example.

Take this simple advice seriously and to heart for your heart. If this isn't getting the results you want; speak to your doctor about medications to treat your risk factors including aiding you with weight loss. **Remember an ounce of prevention is worth a pound of cure!**

How do we put this into practice?
The best made resolutions for a commitment to embracing healthy active living can be thwarted by life stressors, job demands, and unexpected changes to your routine like travel. In this final chapter of bringing, it all together – I provide common **Tipping points** that push people to start making lifestyle changes, **Sticking points** that help people stick with their programs, and conclude by providing **Other tips** to remember. With these, and armed with the new knowledge you have acquired from reading this book, should provide you with the greatest chance of succeeding with your health program long-term.

Risk Factor or Disease	Dietary Changes	+ Exercise Program	Sleep
Diabetes	Low carb	10,000 Steps per day, get heart rate up to sweat	Uninterrupted 7-8 hours
Abdominal Obesity	Low carb	10,000 Steps per day, get heart rate up to sweat	Uninterrupted 7-8 hours
High cholesterol	Low carb Low trans fats MUFA and PUFA over Saturated fats	10,000 Steps per day, get heart rate up to sweat	Uninterrupted 7-8 hours
Fatty Liver	Low Carb	10,000 Steps per day, get heart rate up to sweat	Uninterrupted 7-8 hours
High blood pressure	Diet high in vegetable and Fruit; Watch sodium intake	10,000 Steps per day, get heart rate up to sweat	Uninterrupted 7-8 hours
Heart Attack*	All the above and take medications as prescribed by your doctor.	10,000 Steps per day, get heart rate up to sweat	Uninterrupted 7-8 hours
Stroke or Warning Stroke*	All the above and take all medications as prescribed by your doctor.	10,000 Steps per day, get heart rate up to sweat	Uninterrupted 7-8 hours

Table 3. Recommended Lifestyle Changes per Cardiovascular Concern
*Follow your physicians' advice

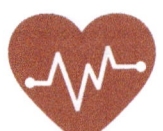

Tipping points

Features in our lives that momentarily jolt us out of our denial that we have adverse health behaviours

Examples from my patients include:

- No longer fitting into a favorite pair of pants, skirt, or blouse
- Family doctor finding "high cholesterol" or borderline diabetes or elevated blood pressure
- Radiologic test showing "fatty liver", atherosclerosis in arteries, old stroke on CT scan or silent heart attack on echo
- Having a heart attack without any warning signs
- Hearing of a loved one, parent or sibling suffering an unexpected heart attack.

Sticking points

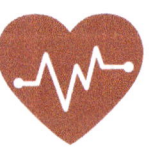

Reasons you are able to adopt and incorporate changes to your eating or activity pattern

Examples from my patients include:

- You have a dog and are obligated to walk the dog two times per day
- You have made a contract with a physician, spouse, friend, or personal trainer to keep up with these changes
- Your insurance premiums go up if you develop a condition like diabetes
- You don't have health insurance and can't "afford" to develop risk factors or heart disease
- You want to be around for your children and be an active grandparent

Other Tips to Remember

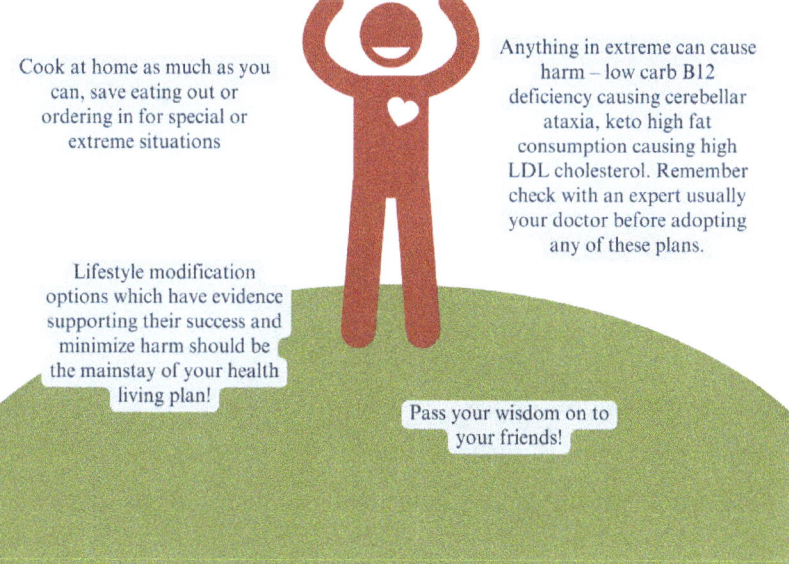

"YoYo is a No No" refers to the adverse effects of adopting different weight loss diets leading to weight cycling, meaning loss of 10 pounds and regain 12.

Intermittent fasting provides a reasonable weight loss approach BUT it is sometimes difficult for people to maintain long-term

Cook at home as much as you can, save eating out or ordering in for special or extreme situations

Anything in extreme can cause harm – low carb B12 deficiency causing cerebellar ataxia, keto high fat consumption causing high LDL cholesterol. Remember check with an expert usually your doctor before adopting any of these plans.

Lifestyle modification options which have evidence supporting their success and minimize harm should be the mainstay of your health living plan!

Pass your wisdom on to your friends!

REFERENCES

Anand, S. S., Samaan, Z., Middleton, C., Irvine, J., Desai, D., Schulze, K. M., Sothiratnam, S., Hussain, F., Shah, B. R., Pare, G., Beyene, J., Lear, S. A., & South Asian Heart Risk Assessment Investigators. (2016). A Digital Health Intervention to Lower Cardiovascular Risk: A Randomized Clinical Trial. JAMA Cardiology, 1(5), 601–606. https://doi.org/10.1001/jamacardio.2016.1035

Dutheil, F., Baker, J. S., Mermillod, M., Cesare, M. D., Vidal, A., Moustafa, F., Pereira, B., & Navel, V. (2020). Shift work, and particularly permanent night shifts, promote dyslipidaemia: A systematic review and meta-analysis. Atherosclerosis, 313, 156–169. https://doi.org/10.1016/j.atherosclerosis.2020.08.01

Kwok, C. S., Kontopantelis, E., Kuligowski, G., Gray, M., Muhyaldeen, A., Gale, C. P., Peat, G. M., Cleator, J., Chew-Graham, C., Loke, Y. K., & Mamas, M. A. (2018). Self-Reported Sleep Duration and Quality and Cardiovascular Disease and Mortality: A Dose-Response Meta-Analysis. Journal of the American Heart Association, 7(15), e008552. https://doi.org/10.1161/JAHA.118.008552

Prochaska, J. O., DiClemente, C. C., & Norcross, J. C. (1992). In search of how people change. Applications to addictive behaviors. The American Psychologist, 47(9), 1102–1114. https://doi.org/10.1037//0003-066x.47.9.1102

www.ingramcontent.com/pod-product-compliance
Lightning Source LLC
Chambersburg PA
CBHW071720020426
42333CB00017B/2335